Department of Health

Report on Health and Social Subjects

50

Folic Acid and the Prevention of Disease

Report of the Committee on Medical
Aspects of Food and Nutrition Policy

London: The Stationery Office

Published with the permission of the Department of Health on behalf of the Controller of Her Majesty's Stationery Office.

First published 2000

ISBN 0 11 322304 8

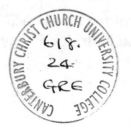

Preface

This report of the Committee on Medical Aspects of Food and Nutrition Policy (COMA) reviews available evidence linking dietary folate and folic acid with human health. It is concerned particularly with the need for adequate intakes of folate at the time of conception to reduce the risk of a pregnancy being affected by a neural tube defect (NTD), of which spina bifida is a common form.

Almost a decade ago it was shown that folic acid supplements taken at the time of conception could reduce the incidence of NTDs by two-thirds. Over the last decade, annual numbers of NTD births in the United Kingdom have been declining but, to an uncertain extent, this has been due to detection and termination of affected pregnancies with the attendant costs and distress. A government-sponsored campaign to encourage women who might become pregnant to take supplements of folic acid has been of some success but many pregnancies are unplanned and by the time a woman knows she is pregnant it may be too late for folic acid to be effective.

This is the background to calls for fortification of food with folic acid, as has been instituted in the United States. This proposal needs rigorous examination as there is a possibility that large amounts of folic acid in the diet might be deleterious for people in the community who have undiagnosed pernicious anaemia. The Committee has identified a level of fortification that would provide significant benefit in reducing the incidence of pregnancies affected by NTD without exposing any section of the population to risks. There is reason to hope that such an increase in dietary folate would also be beneficial in reducing the incidence of cardiovascular disease throughout the population, but the Committee considered that the evidence for this was not yet sufficiently complete to justify fortification simply for that purpose.

The Committee is concerned with the scientific aspects of nutrition; it is not our business to develop policy. We have to be aware of policy issues to ensure that we review the relevant areas of scientific knowledge and appraise an appropriate range of options. The formulation of policy is the responsibility of ministers and requires consideration of such matters as legal and regulatory issues, social and political priorities and economic implications, which are outside the Committee's remit.

It is a pleasure to record the Committee's thanks to the members of the Working Group, its superb secretariat, and all those who have helped it in what has been a large and complex task. We all have reason to be grateful for the commitment to the public good of the scientists who have so unstintingly given of their time and expertise.

PROFESSOR SIR JOHN GRIMLEY EVANS
Chairman, Committee on Medical Aspects of Food and Nutrition Policy

Contents

Committee on Medical Aspects of Food and Nutrition Policy

Chairman

Sir Kenneth Calman
(up to April 1998)

Chief Medical Officer for England

Professor Sir John Grimley Evans
(from September 1998)

Division of Clinical Geratology,
Nuffield Department of Clinical
Medicine, University of Oxford

Members

Professor P Aggett

Head of Lancashire Postgraduate
School of Medicine and Health,
University of Central Lancashire

Dr S Bingham

Deputy Director, MRC Dunn
Nutrition Unit, Cambridge

Professor G Fowler

Professor Emeritus of General
Practice, University of Oxford

Professor A A Jackson

Professor of Human Nutrition,
University of Southampton

Professor W P T James

Director Rowett Research Institute,
Aberdeen (until June 1999)

Professor M Marmot

Professor of Epidemiology and Public
Health, University College Medical
School, London

Professor D P Richardson

Nestlé UK Limited, Croydon, Surrey

Dr P Troop
(until September 1999)

Regional Director of Public Health,
Anglia and Oxford, Milton Keynes

Dr A F Williams

Senior Lecturer and Consultant in
Neonatal Paediatrics, St George's
Hospital, London

Assessors

Professor L Donaldson (from October 1998)	Chief Medical Officer for England
Dr H Campbell	Chief Medical Officer, DHSS Northern Ireland
Professor Sir David Carter	Chief Medical Officer, Department of Health, Scottish Office
Dr R Hall	Chief Medical Officer, Welsh Office
Dr A Peatfield	Medical Research Council
Mr G Podger	Ministry of Agriculture, Fisheries and Food
Dr E Rubery (until July 1999)	Department of Health
Ms L Stockley (until April 1999)	Health Education Authority
Ms K Peploe (from October 1999)	Health Education Authority

Secretariat from the Department of Health

Dr S Reddy (Scientific)	(from February 1998)
Dr A Redfern (Scientific)	(until January 1999)
Dr P Clarke (Medical)	(retired August 1998)
Mr B Wenlock (Scientific)	(from September 1998)
Professor M Wiseman (Medical)	(until July 1999)
Miss Yemi Fagun (Administrative)	(from June 1998)
Miss C Dick (Scientific)	(from April 1999)
Miss S Kunar (Scientific)	(from April 1999)
Miss S Collaco (Administrative)	

Committee on Medical Aspects of Food and Nutrition Policy

Working Group on the Nutritional Status of the Population (disbanded in October 1998)

Chairman

Professor P Aggett	Head of Lancashire Postgraduate School of Medicine and Health, University of Central Lancashire

Members

Dr D Buss (d. 29 August 1998)	Independent Nutrition Consultant, Hampshire
Professor Sir John Grimley Evans	Division of Clinical Geratology, Nuffield Department of Clinical Medicine, University of Oxford
Professor A A Jackson	Professor of Human Nutrition, University of Southampton
Dr A Prentice	Director, MRC Human Nutrition Research, Cambridge
Professor A Shenkin	Department of Clinical Chemistry, University of Liverpool

Assessor

Mr W J Scriven (from 1997)	Ministry of Agriculture, Fisheries and Food

Secretariat from the Department of Health

Dr P C Clarke (Medical) (retired August 1998)
Dr A Redfern (Scientific)
Professor M Wiseman (Medical)

Committee on Medical Aspects of Food and Nutrition Policy

Subgroup (now Working Group) on Folic Acid

Chairman

Prof Sir John Grimley Evans   Division of Clinical Geratology, Nuffield Department of Clinical Medicine, University of Oxford

Members

Professor P Aggett   Head of Lancashire School of Postgraduate Medicine and Health, University of Central Lancashire

Professor A V Hoffbrand   Department of Haematology, Royal Free Hospital, London

Professor A A Jackson   Department of Human Nutrition, University of Southampton

Professor A Malcolm   Chief Executive, Institute of Biology, London

Dr E H Reynolds   Bethlem Royal Hospital and Maudsley Hospital, London

Professor J M Scott   Department of Biochemistry, University of Dublin, Ireland

Professor M J Seller   Division of Medical and Molecular Genetics, The Guy's, Kings & St Thomas' School of Medicine, London

Professor N Wald   Department of Environmental and Preventive Medicine, St Bartholomew's Hospital, London

Assessors

Ms S Oldreive (until July 1998) Ministry of Agriculture, Fisheries and Food, London

Ms H Lee (from July 1998) Ministry of Agriculture, Fisheries and Food, London

Secretariat from the Department of Health

Dr P C Clarke (Medical) (retired August 1998)
Dr S Reddy (Scientific) (from July 1998)
Dr A Redfern (Scientific) (until January 1999)
Professor M Wiseman (Medical) (until July 1999)
Miss S Collaco (Administrative)
Mrs B Hegan (Scientific) (from January-April 1999)
Miss S Kunar (Scientific) (from April 1999)
Miss C Dick (Scientific) (from April 1999)

Experts invited to consider homocysteine and CVD

Dr C Bates MRC, Human Nutrition Research, Cambridge

Dr R Clarke University of Oxford

Professor I Graham Charlemont Clinic, Dublin

Professor M Marmot University College/Middlesex Medical Schools, London

Dr V Press Representing the British Heart Foundation

Dr P Whincup Royal Free Hospital School of Medicine, London

Professor J Wraith Royal Manchester Children's Hospital

Experts invited to consider Review of Dietary Reference Values for Folate

Dr C Bates MRC, Human Nutrition Research, Cambridge

Dr C Schorah University of Leeds

Dr D Bender University College, London

Acknowledgements

COMA is grateful to the following, who provided written submissions to the Working Group.

Food and Drink Federation	London
Kellogg's Company	Manchester
The Maternity Alliance	London
National Association of Millers and Bakers	London
Royal College of Obstetricians and Gynaecologists	London
Safeway Stores plc	Hayes, Middlesex
Mr David Godfrey*	Roche Products Ltd
Dr Paul Finglas/ Dr Anthony J Wright*	Diet, Health & Consumer Science Division, Institute of Food Research, Norwich
Ms Lucy Thorpe*	Health Education Authority
Dr Michael Murphy*	Imperial Cancer Research Fund General Practice Research Group, Oxford

* Submissions were requested by COMA

Overview

A.   Historical background

A.1   Severe deficiency of the B vitamin folate produces a type of anaemia that was first recognised as the "anaemia of poverty" in Bombay in 1931. Since then it has become apparent that relatively low folate intakes, common in Western populations (not merely the gross deficiency necessary to cause anaemia) may have other important effects on health. During the 1960s, it was suggested that the risk of a woman bearing a child with a neural tube defect (NTD) might be affected by her folate intake, and in 1991 dietary supplements of folic acid were shown by a randomised trial to reduce the risk of NTDs. Folic acid is an artificial form of the naturally occurring vitamin folate. More recently, research has linked low folate intake to raised levels of homocysteine in the blood, and possibly to an increased risk of occlusive vascular disease and neuropsychiatric disorders (Section 1.1).

A.2   During the 1990s, public health policy with regard to preventing NTDs aimed to ensure that women of childbearing age were aware of the importance of acquiring sufficient folic acid and folate in the diet at the time of conception to minimise the risk of NTDs in their offspring. Over that period, dietary supplements of folic acid, some licensed medicinal products, and foods fortified with folic acid became more widely available. However, it is apparent that many women still become pregnant while consuming insufficient folate to minimise the risk of a pregnancy affected by NTD. In the UK, as in the USA, there have been calls for more active public policy, including food fortification, to address this. It was therefore timely for COMA to undertake a review of the links between folates, including folic acid, and disease.

B.   Interpretation of remit

The responsibility for decisions on public health policy rests with Government. In order to exercise this responsibility, Government obtains advice on possible policies, and their implications, from various sources. Advice on the medical and scientific aspects of nutrition is one major factor in developing public health policy, but others usually also need to be considered in reaching a final decision. Although our expertise and remit are in medical and scientific issues, in providing our advice we have borne in mind the existing policy and regulatory context as it has been explained to us. We were also conscious of ethical issues raised by the mandatory fortification of food, particularly where possible risks of fortification might fall to a group of the population different from that receiving the benefits. Finally, we have not considered economic considerations to be within our remit, although they will have to be taken into account in the formulation of public policy.

C.   Folate, folic acid and NTD

C.1   Folate is a generic term for compounds that have a common vitamin activity, and includes folic acid. Natural folates are compounds that occur naturally in foods with the same vitamin function as its artificial form, folic acid, which is used in dietary supplements and for fortification of foods (Sections 2.1 and 2.2). Total folate intake of an individual comprises natural folates and folic acid consumed either as a fortificant or in the form of dietary supplements. Folic acid is more stable in foods and is better absorbed than natural folates. In the British diet, the main sources of folate are cereals and vegetables, and a significant proportion of this is obtained through fortification, especially of breakfast cereals. The average total folate intake per head of population in Britain in 1998 was about 250 µg/day (Section 3.4).

C.2   The original suggestion that folate intake might influence the risk of NTD was based on observational data relating to maternal blood levels and on early intervention studies (Section 5.1, 5.2 and 5.3). In 1991, the Medical Research Council (MRC) Vitamin Trial reported that a significant reduction in the recurrence of NTD had been obtained by a daily dietary supplement of 4 mg (4000 µg) of folic acid in women at high risk (para 1.1.2). A later study reported that first occurrence of NTD could also be prevented by daily supplements containing 800 µg of folic acid (Table 5.2). The predicted efficacy of doses of 400 µg daily was based on the results of earlier intervention studies. This is the level of supplementation recommended by the majority of nations, including the UK, giving official guidance to women of childbearing age with no previous history of pregnancies affected by NTD. A study from Ireland indicated that women taking daily supplements of 400 µg attained blood levels of folate associated with a low risk of NTD pregnancy (para 5.3.5). In China, a non-randomised study found that a periconceptional supplement of 400 µg daily significantly reduced the frequency of NTDs in both high- and low-incidence districts. Against a daily background intake in the UK of around 200 µg, at the time the earlier studies were performed, the recommended extra intake of 400 µg implies a target total daily intake of 600 µg or more for women exposed to the possibility of becoming pregnant.

C.3   Because NTDs affect only a small minority of women, even of those with low folate intakes, it seemed possible that the risk of NTD was influenced by a genetic factor, which could in part be overcome by extra folic acid (Section 2.5). There is now some direct evidence for this but, more important, there is evidence of a graded relationship between intake of folic acid/folate and folate status on the one hand and risk of NTD on the other (Section 5.2). From the perspective of public health policy, there is no practical means at present whereby population screening could be effective through identifying a subgroup of women with particular need for folic acid supplements to prevent NTDs in their children. In contrast, there is evidence that increasing average folic acid intake will confer a worthwhile preventive effect (Section 5.3).

C.4   The education campaigns conducted since 1995 have had a substantial effect in increasing the number of women aware of the link between folic acid

2

and the risk of NTD. While in 1995 only 9% of women of childbearing age were aware of the need for women who might become pregnant to take extra folic acid, in 1998 the proportion had risen to 49% (Annex 2). A policy of advising periconceptional supplements of folic acid to be taken by women planning pregnancies may have a limited impact, as roughly a half of pregnancies are unplanned. Such education can therefore have only a limited effect. With current fortification practices, it would be difficult with a normal diet to achieve an intake equivalent to 400 μg/day of extra folic acid. There is also evidence that the bioavailability of naturally occurring folates is lower than that of folic acid added to foods or in dietary supplements (para 3.2.2). NTDs arise very early in gestation; by the time a woman realises she is pregnant it is usually too late to prevent an NTD by taking supplements (Section 4.1). For these reasons it has been suggested that the most effective way of reducing the incidence of NTD would be to fortify the food supply with folic acid so that even women with unplanned pregnancies would be less likely than at present to have offspring with NTD.

C.5   The mechanism for the effect of folic acid in reducing the risk of NTD is not clear. The most likely explanation is that it overcomes genetically determined defects in folate metabolism that interfere with normal neural tube development. One other hypothesis is that it might decrease the likelihood of an affected pregnancy surviving, and there is some concern that folic acid supplementation could be associated with higher risk of fetal death. However, the generally accepted explanation for this is that folic acid might initially permit the survival of affected or non-viable pregnancies to a point when they are recognised as spontaneous abortions (Section 4.4).

D.   **Possible other benefits and hazards**

D.1   A proposal for general food fortification to prevent neural tube defects requires consideration of possible benefits and hazards not only to women of childbearing age but also to other sections of the population. Important possible benefits include a reduction in the risk of cardiovascular disease (especially strokes and heart attacks) (Chapter 6) and of mood disorders and dementia (Chapter 7). Possible risks are an increase in neurological disorders in people with undiagnosed deficiency of vitamin B_{12} and interactions between folic acid and some medications (Chapter 7).

D.2   It has been known for some time that people with rare genetic disorders that greatly increase the level of homocysteine in their blood have a high risk of cardiovascular diseases (CVD) such as strokes and heart attacks (para 6.1.2). More recently, it has been demonstrated that in otherwise healthy people, more modest elevations of plasma levels of homocysteine are associated with higher risk of CVD. Studies have shown that low intakes of folate are an important cause of raised plasma homocysteine in the general population, and increasing folate intake can reduce plasma homocysteine (paras 6.1.2 and 6.1.3). This raises the possibility that a substantial proportion of the UK population might reduce their risk of CVD by increasing their intake of folate/folic acid. As cardiovascular

3

disease is the single greatest cause of mortality in the UK, the public health implications are substantial. However, although there are several indications that the relationship is causal, confirmation requires an intervention study and evidence from randomised trials showing that reducing homocysteine levels reduces CVD incidence; no such trials have yet been reported (Sections 6.3 and 6.4).

D.3   Several studies have demonstrated poor folate status in people with a variety of neuropsychiatric conditions. It is not clear from observational studies whether the poorer status is a result of the mental state, or *vice versa*, or a combination of the two. Some, but not all, studies of folate supplementation have demonstrated benefit, but these should be interpreted with caution because of flaws in experimental design. Nevertheless, if such a relationship were confirmed, the implications would be substantial (Chapter 7).

D.4   The metabolism of folate is interrelated with that of another vitamin, vitamin B_{12}. Some people, mainly vegans, may have a dietary deficiency of vitamin B_{12}, usually mild, but there is also a group of mainly older people who develop an inability to absorb the vitamin (Sections 8.1 and 8.2). This is either due to a condition known as pernicious anaemia, where there is failure of synthesis of gastric intrinsic factor necessary for the absorption of vitamin B_{12}, or to a milder form of atrophic gastritis with reduced production of intrinsic factor. Other less common diseases of the stomach or intestine may cause failure of absorption of vitamin B_{12}. Deficiency of vitamin B_{12} has two main effects: it can cause an anaemia identical to that of folate deficiency; and it can cause damage to the nerves and the spinal cord, leading to severe disability. The latter is seen only in severe deficiency of vitamin B_{12}, which is associated with pernicious anaemia and not milder forms accompanying atrophic gastritis or veganism, and is very rare in folate deficiency. The anaemia usually appears first but, unlike the nerve damage, treatment with folic acid can delay or prevent it. A general increase in folate and folic acid intake in the population might therefore change the clinical presentation of vitamin B_{12} deficiency. There have also been anecdotal reports that high intakes of folic acid (more than 1 mg per day) might hasten the onset of neurological damage in people whose deficiency of vitamin B_{12} has not been recognised. There is anxiety that such an effect, though not reported, might also occur at lower levels, particularly if supplementation is prolonged. However, there is no conclusive evidence that this effect occurs, and it has not been reported at folic acid intakes of less than 1 mg/day. Nevertheless, it is important that there should be no unnecessary delay in diagnosing vitamin B_{12} deficiency, whatever the intake of folate and folic acid, particularly in older people and vegans.

D.5   A further concern is that an increase in folic acid intake might lead to some patients taking anti-epileptic treatment needing to change dosage, but regular monitoring and adjustment of such medication is already established as part of good clinical practice (Section 7.4). There is no evidence to support the theoretical concern that folic acid supplementation might interfere with the efficiency of antifolate chemotherapeutic agents such as methotrexate.

4

E.   Implications of fortification

E.1   For the reasons given above, our considerations focused on the possible effectiveness and implications of fortifying foods with folic acid. The target group for whom benefits are certain (pregnant women and their children) is different from that on whom possible hazards might fall (mainly older people with undiagnosed vitamin B_{12} deficiency). On the other hand, the latter group might also benefit considerably from reduced CVD risk. The likelihood of hazards and benefits in this older group is less certain than the benefits in women of childbearing age. However, one result of a fortification policy would be that all sectors of society would be exposed. There is little information on the possible effect of higher folate and folic acid intake amongst other groups such as children and young men, although there is no *prima facie* reason to expect any adverse effects. In some countries (for instance the United States, which has already introduced mandatory fortification of grain products with folic acid) observational data could become available. There is good evidence that, for a number of years, over one-third of all adults in the USA have habitually taken daily supplements that contain 400 µg of folic acid. No adverse effects have been reported as a result of this practice.

E.2   Unlike the situation with the use of supplements, with fortification the dose to individuals cannot be tightly controlled. It is therefore important to examine the likely range of intakes by target groups and by potentially vulnerable groups for any given level of fortification, and for a variety of number and types of foods fortified. We selected models involving fortification of flour (mainly but not exclusively as bread) and breakfast cereals (many of which are already fortified with folic acid) because of their near universal consumption, and the relatively narrow variation in consumption levels (Annexes 6 and 7). However, we are aware that even with the excellent data that formed the basis of these models, they could not adequately take account of the day-to-day variation in the consumption of breads and breakfast cereals, or of the possible technical difficulties in achieving a uniform level of folic acid in the food supply. The fortification levels used in the modelling are for the amount of folic acid per 100 g of flour in the finished/final product as consumed (not simply added to flour at source) and so losses through processing and storage will need to be considered.

E.3   Not all NTDs are due to folate deficiency, and whatever policy is adopted, some will continue to occur. Even with relatively high intakes of folic acid, a maximum of around one-third of NTDs can be expected still to occur (Table 9.1). Some people might question the propriety of manipulating the diet of the entire nation to compensate for the small number of women who do not follow well-publicised advice to take folic acid supplements if exposed to the possibility of becoming pregnant. Not all women, however, are aware of the significance of the advice and many pregnancies are unintended. A civilised society accepts a duty to protect its vulnerable members. The consequences of the inevitable occasional failures of even the most assiduous supplementation policy fall most heavily on the children born with severe disabilities. A further consequence is the contribution, often substantial, to the costs of their care made by the general community.

E.4   An appropriate policy would be, for women of childbearing age to attain the current recommendation of an extra 400 μg of folic acid per day in addition to normal dietary folate intake, while ensuring that no-one was exposed to intakes high enough to cause adverse effects. In particular, the possibility of neurological damage (neuropathy) in people who are deficient in vitamin B_{12} should be borne in mind. The British National Formulary (para 8.2.2) cautions that folic acid should not be given alone in the treatment of pernicious anaemia and other vitamin B_{12} deficiency states because it may precipitate the onset of subacute combined degeneration of the spinal cord. There have been no conclusive reports that neurological damage occurs below a daily folic acid intake of 2 mg (2000 μg), although some clinicians remain concerned over the possibility. An upper daily intake of 1 mg (1000 μg) therefore seems to offer a wide margin of safety for this vulnerable group, who are mainly over 50 years of age.

E.5   It is likely that many conceptions with NTD abort spontaneously in the first trimester, but about a half of these are due to chromosomal abnormalities almost certainly not related to folate status. The number of pregnancies affected by NTD that pass into the second trimester is unknown, but estimates for the UK range from 600 to 1200 per year. A number of these abort spontaneously and a further proportion are terminated around 20 weeks of gestation following antenatal detection (Annex 5). There are around 90 births each year of children affected by NTD in England and Wales and around 60 in Scotland and 15 in Northern Ireland (Annex 5). A daily dose of 400 μg of extra folic acid would be expected to reduce the incidence of pregnancies affected by NTD by about a half. Observational data suggest that a lower dose of an extra 200 μg daily would produce a reduction of about 30% (about two-thirds of the maximum attainable effect) in the number of affected pregnancies and so prevent a substantial number of affected pregnancies annually. It is not possible to estimate what proportion of these would have progressed to term. However, it is clear that extra folic acid would avoid much of the trauma and distress of antenatal diagnosis of affected pregnancies and consequent termination of wanted pregnancies. With current incidence, we estimate that around 38 NTD births could be prevented by a daily dose of 200 μg of extra folic acid in the diets of women becoming pregnant. These calculations are based in part on data relating folate status to NTD risk, and folate intake to folate status (Table 9.1). These data, though recent, are not extensive. The calculations are also based on the results of the MRC Vitamin Study, performed around 10 years ago. However rates of NTD at birth have declined over this period and folate intakes by pregnant women have increased, so it is not known whether the proportionate effect of folic acid supplementation would now be the same.

E.6   Apart from the effects of reducing the risk of NTD, and, possibly, altering the presentation of vitamin B_{12} deficiency, and the dosage of medication required by people with epilepsy, there are other implications of a fortification policy in particular, the possible benefit in reducing the risk of CVD. First, however, the evidence that increasing the intake of folate/folic acid would reduce the incidence of CVD is currently not conclusive, and requires confirmation. Universal fortification would make it more difficult in the future to conduct a study in the

6

UK into the role of folic acid in preventing CVD, although such research could be carried out elsewhere where fortification does not occur. There is no suggestion that increasing folate or folic acid might increase risk of CVD, and so the outcome of fortification would only be expected to be either neutral or advantageous in respect of risk of CVD (while the effects on NTD are clearly established). The possible benefits in neuropsychiatric disorders are more speculative at present.

E.7   Second, a policy of universal fortification, unlike voluntary dietary supplementation, would not allow the element of individual consent to the exposure. There is no universal agreement on when it is appropriate for other factors to override personal discretion. However, the protection of vulnerable groups is one feature of civilised societies, and securing the health of children (both before and after birth) might be seen as a reasonable responsibility of society as a whole. In some countries, such as the Netherlands, food fortification is restricted, while in the USA statutory fortification of foods with folic acid is already in force. The statutory fortification of a number of foods with nutrients to protect public health is a long-standing and current practice in many countries, including the UK, as is the voluntary addition of some nutrients. There is a balance of advantage and disadvantage in following either of these paths. Even in the absence of health risks to people exposed to fortified food, a change to established practice can be expected to raise public concerns that need to be carefully considered.

E.8   It is worth noting that the food supply is already voluntarily and variably fortified with folic acid in the absence of statutory regulation, and better control of the exposure of the population might be advantageous. For instance, people who are potentially at risk of neuropathy might already be consuming fortified breakfast cereals unaware of any possible risks. It has been estimated in a small study in the USA that 1.2% of people aged 60 and over might have undetected pernicious anaemia with vitamin B_{12} deficiency and so might be at risk of adverse effects from inadvertent high folic acid intake (para 8.2.5). Food fortification with folic acid could be controlled in relation both to the levels of fortification and to those foods that are fortified. In addition, even if suboptimal folate intakes in the population facilitate the detection of vitamin B_{12} deficiency, it would be perverse to maintain the present situation for that reason. Decisions on whether or not to require the food industry to add folic acid to foods need to take account of all these factors, and in particular what is deemed at the time to be an appropriate balance between the roles of individuals and of the state. Any intervention by the Government needs to be proportionate to the situation.

F   **Options for action**

F.1   The prevailing content of folate/folic acid in the British household food supply (an average of 250 µg/day) is below that necessary to minimise risk of NTD in women of childbearing age, which can be achieved by an additional intake of 400 µg/day. In addition, a number of people in other sections of the population, in particular older people, do not consume folate/folic acid at a level estimated to meet their requirements, based on existing Dietary Reference Values

(DRV), and biochemical markers of folate status are also low in this group. Higher folate intakes can be achieved either by individual decisions to take dietary supplements of folic acid or eat foods rich in natural folates or fortified with folic acid, or by more generally fortifying the food supply to increase intakes in the population as a whole. The most recent estimate of total folate intake in women of childbearing age is around 200 µg/day (Table A7.1). An increase of 400 µg/day of folic acid would reduce the risk of NTDs substantially (by an estimated 47-53%), and this level of 600 µg/day could not be reasonably achieved without fortification or by more widespread use of supplements. The most appropriate staple foods for fortification would be flour and breakfast cereals because of their near universal consumption and relatively narrow variability of consumption in the population. If universal fortification were to be adopted, an intake of at least 600 µg/day of folic acid by all women of childbearing age could not be achieved without exposing large numbers of older people, aged 50 and over, to intakes above 1 mg/day (Table A7.2).

F.2   After careful consideration of possible benefits and hazards, we have appraised some options for action based on a modelling exercise to estimate expected intakes in different age groups, at various levels of fortification of flour. The options balance the possible benefits to younger women of protecting them from NTD conceptions, against possible adverse effects such as neuropathy, especially in older people who might have vitamin B_{12} deficiency. A range of levels of fortification was chosen (para 9.5.9). We have assumed target levels of fortification such that the level is precisely maintained in the food supply over a reasonable period of time. To ensure that levels do not fall below such a minimum, manufacturers usually add more nutrients (overage) than necessary to take account of losses during processing and storage. However, if such an overage were used in fortifying foods with folic acid, this would exceed the target level, and people would be exposed to higher than expected levels. Unfortunately, the degree of overage is highly variable, and no research has been done on the ability of industry to deliver a target (as opposed to the minimum) level (para 9.5.10). Such uncertainty argues for caution in translating the concept into a safe and effective policy. Whichever option is chosen, there should be continued monitoring of rates of NTD occurrence, and clinical vigilance with regard to older people, with the aim of early detection of vitamin B_{12} deficiency. In addition, there should be regular monitoring of fortification levels in bread and other products containing flour. The options for action suggested below are based on data available at the present time and should not be regarded as permanent solutions. Any policy should be reviewed in the future in the light of changes in the prevailing situation, particularly with regard to improvements in methodology of folate analysis and the emerging scientific knowledge on bioavailability of natural folates and folic acid from foods.

F.3   The expected benefits of different options (Section 9.6) appraised by us are summarised below.

Option 1   *Continue or intensify education programme without universal fortification*

The success of the folic acid campaign in raising the awareness (Annex 2) of women planning to become pregnant with regard to the importance of increasing folic acid intakes argues for the continuation, and possibly intensification, of the programme. Monitoring of rates of NTD and changes in the uptake of termination options should provide the basis for evaluating the effectiveness of the education programme. This option, taken alone, is unlikely to increase folic acid intake amongst the proportion of women whose pregnancies are unplanned, or to benefit the group of older people whose folate/folic acid intakes remain low. However, this option is not exclusive of other options, and there would be advantage in continuing existing education whatever other policies may also be adopted.

Option 2   *Fortification at 140 μg/100 g of flour*

- The average intake of folic acid of women aged 16-45 years would increase by 117 μg/day, leading to an average total folate intake of 321 μg/day (Table 9.1).

- Approximately 0.7% of women in this age group would have total folate intakes in excess of 600 μg/day.

- It is estimated that 23 NTD-affected births per year would be prevented (Table 9.1).

- Approximately 0.1% of people aged over 50 years would be exposed to levels of folic acid intake greater than 1 mg/day (Table A7.2).

Option 3   *Fortification at 200 μg/100 g of flour*

- The average intake of folic acid of women aged 16-45 years would increase by 167 μg/day, leading to a total folate intake of 371 μg/day (Table 9.1).

- Approximately 2.8% of women in this age group would have total folate intakes in excess of 600 μg/day.

- It is estimated that 32 NTD-affected births per year would be prevented (Table 9.1).

- Approximately 0.2% of people aged over 50 years would be exposed to levels of folic acid intake greater than 1 mg/day (Table A7.2).

Option 4   *Fortification at 240 μg/100 g of flour*

- The average intake of folic acid of women aged 16-45 years would increase by 201 μg/day, leading to a total folate intake of 405 μg/day (Table 9.1).

- Approximately 7% of women in this age group would have total folate intakes in excess of 600 µg/day.

- It is estimated that 38 NTD-affected births per year would be prevented (Table 9.1).

- Approximately 0.6% of people aged over 50 years would be exposed to levels of folic acid intake greater than 1 mg/day (Table A7.2).

Option 5 *Fortification at 280 µg/100 g of flour*

- The average intake of folic acid of women aged 16-45 years would increase by 234 µg/day, leading to a total folate intake of 438 µg/day (Table 9.1).

- Approximately 13% of women in this age group would have total folate intakes in excess of 600 µg/day.

- It is estimated that 39 NTD-affected births per year would be prevented (Table 9.1).

- Approximately 1.5% of people aged over 50 years would be exposed to levels of folic acid intake greater than 1 mg/day (Table A7.2).

Option 6 *Fortification at 420 µg/100 g of flour*

- The average intake of folic acid of women aged 16-45 years would increase by 351 µg/day, leading to a total folate intake of 555 µg/day (Table 9.1).

- Approximately 40% of women in this age group would have total folate intakes in excess of 600 µg/day.

- It is estimated that 42 NTD-affected births per year would be prevented (Table 9.1).

- Approximately 9% of people aged over 50 years would be exposed to levels of folic acid intake greater than 1 mg/day (Table A7.2).

Option 7 *Combined fortification with folic acid and vitamin B$_{12}$*

In order to minimise the possibility of vitamin B$_{12}$ deficiency, particularly in older people, the possibility and practicality of fortifying foods with vitamin B$_{12}$ might be considered. There is no evidence of toxicity of vitamin B$_{12}$ and, moreover, it has recently been shown that combined supplementation with both vitamins was efficacious in lowering circulating homocysteine levels (para 8.2.6). At present, there is inadequate information on the amount of vitamin B$_{12}$ that would be required to prevent deficiency in the population, especially in those with pernicious anaemia. Although there is no formal evidence of toxicity from vitamin B_{12}, any exposure of the whole population to levels many times their usual intake or requirements should be considered with particular caution.

G   Technical issues

We have modelled the likely exposures of various population groups on the basis of different levels of fortification of flour with folic acid, and assuming no change in the intake of folic acid from other sources. A particular source of folic acid is breakfast cereals. However, as there are concerns not only about low, but also about excessive intake of folic acid, it is important to the eventual outcome that current levels of fortification of breakfast cereals do not change substantially. Any such change would make an important difference to the numbers of people exposed to different levels of folic acid, and so also to the balance of risk against benefit in the population as a whole. Consideration will need to be given as to whether the levels of folic acid in breakfast cereals should be subject to some degree of control. Furthermore, these calculations are based on a precise addition of folic acid to flour at the target level, but manufacturers will have to ensure that the target levels are maintained in flour products as consumed. However, for technical reasons, there is likely to be variation around this, and any decisions should take account of the ability of manufacturers not only to avoid unexpectedly low, but also undesirably high levels of folic acid in flour and its products.

H   Conclusion

On scientific, medical and public health grounds, the Committee concluded that universal folic acid fortification of flour at 240 μg/100 g in food products as consumed would have a significant effect in preventing NTD-affected conceptions and births without resulting in unacceptably high intakes in any group of the population.

1. Introduction

1.1 Background

1.1.1 In 1931, Dr Lucy Wills demonstrated cure of macrocytic anaemia in pregnancy by a factor present in yeast. In 1944, the factor was isolated from spinach and the name folate was used because it was derived from leafy vegetables. It subsequently emerged that the factor was a vitamin and comprised a group of naturally occurring derivatives of pteroyl glutamic acid (folic acid). Other rich food sources include oranges and some other fruits and vegetables, as well as yeast extract and liver. Several derivatives of pteroyl glutamic acid have metabolic activity, and this has contributed to the difficulties in defining and measuring the total folate content of foods and of biological materials (Annex 3). This is one of the reasons why folates have only recently been included in analyses of diet and nutrition surveys. These problems have also made it difficult to set population Dietary Reference Values (DRV) (para 3.1.4). Recent advances in laboratory techniques mean that research into the physiological and pathological significance of differences in folate status are now more soundly based.

1.1.2 Since 1964 it has been recognised that folate status might affect a woman's risk of having a baby with NTD. However, early evidence was non-specific and inconclusive. In the early 1980s, studies on recurrence of NTD in women who already had an affected infant suggested that folic acid pre-conceptionally and during the first weeks of pregnancy had a preventive effect, but the results were confounded by the presence of other nutrients in the multivitamin supplement, which also included folic acid. The MRC Vitamin Study in 1991 demonstrated the benefits of folic acid supplementation in a large group of women. A total of 1817 women at high risk of an NTD-affected pregnancy because of a previous affected pregnancy were allocated at random to one of four groups to receive folic acid (at the high dose of 4 mg daily), other multivitamins, multivitamins with folic acid or placebo containing ferrous sulphate and di-calcium phosphate. The study design was factorial, which meant that around half of the subjects were taking folic acid supplements, with or without other multivitamins. The women who received folic acid experienced a significantly lower relative risk of pregnancy affected by NTD, at 0.28 (95% confidence interval (CI 0.12-0.71), compared with 0.80 (95% CI 0.32-1.72) in women who received no folic acid[1].

1.1.3 The UK Government Health Departments first issued guidance about folic acid and the prevention of recurrence of neural tube defects in 1991[2]. In response to a report from experts[3], the guidance was expanded to cover the prevention of first-time NTDs. The conclusions of this report are presented in Annex 1 and include the recommendation that all women planning a pregnancy should take 400 µg of folic acid as a daily supplement. Against a background dietary folate intake of the order of 200 µg, this implies a recommended total daily intake of 600 µg. This is within the range of recommendations offered by other national governments, which vary from a total intake (all sources) of 400 µg to a supplement of 1000 µg (1 mg) daily[4]. Following the Health Education Authority's Folic Acid Campaign, background awareness among women of childbearing age of the need to take folic acid to reduce the risk of NTD rose from 9% in 1995 to 49% in 1998, while prompted awareness rose from 51% in 1995 to 89% in 1998 (Annex 2). Although there has been an encouraging increase in the proportion of women reporting that they took folic acid when planning a pregnancy, women from lower social classes were less likely to take folic acid supplements. In addition, between 30% and 50% of all conceptions in England and Wales are unintended[5,6] and some women of reproductive age are not reached by the campaign.

1.1.4   More recently, it has been found that folate status is also related to the risk of vascular disease, possibly via its effect on homocysteine levels[7,8]. In a report on The Nutritional Aspects of Cardiovascular Disease in 1994, the Committee on the Medical Aspects of Food and Nutrition Policy noted this association, but the evidence was then inconclusive and folate status was not specifically considered[9]. Since then, considerable data have emerged confirming the association between raised homocysteine levels and the increased risk of cardiovascular disease. It remains to be demonstrated whether reducing homocysteine, for example by increasing folic acid intake, actually reduces the risk of CVD.

1.2   Terms of reference

The Government is advised on matters relating to diet, nutrition and health by the Committee on Medical Aspects of Food and Nutrition Policy (COMA) through the Chief Medical Officer. This Committee had set up a Working Group on the Nutritional Status of the Population[+] with the following terms of reference:-

"To review the dietary intakes and nutritional status of the population with regard to folic acid and the nutrients currently statutorily added to flour and yellow fats;

To consider mechanisms, including fortification of foods, for the maintenance of adequate nutritional status and evaluation of their safety and effectiveness;

To make recommendations on the above;

To advise on a programme of work to review the dietary intakes and nutritional status of the population with regard to other nutrients."

[+] This group was disbanded in October 1998 and the responsibilities of the group have been transferred to the main committee.

Established, in the first instance, to review issues relating to the fortification of foods, this Working Group also considered nutritional matters referred to it by COMA as they emerged from the programme of National Diet and Nutrition Surveys[10,11]. Since 1992, several new questions had arisen concerning folic acid and the prevention of disease, and this Working Group of COMA agreed to set up a Subgroup on Folic Acid with terms of reference:

> "To consider the dietary intakes and nutritional status of the population in regard to folic acid with particular reference to its contribution in preventing disease, and to make recommendations."

The 1992 report on Neural Tube Defects from the Department of Health had not been prepared under the auspices of COMA, and it was considered appropriate to assess the broad nutritional issues surrounding folic acid and its relationship to disease.

1.3   Meetings of the Working Group

The meeting on 2 October 1996 was the first of six meetings of the Working Group, and a call was made for submissions. On 24 September 1997, a meeting was held between the members of the Working Group and additional invited experts to consider the nature of the relationship between folate status, folic acid intake and vascular disease. On 12 February 1999, a meeting was held between the Working Group and additional invited experts to consider whether there was a need to review the DRV for folate in the light of emerging evidence on the effect of folate on homocysteine levels. COMA considered the report from the Working Group on 28 April 1999.

1.4   Consideration of evidence

The evidence relating folate and folic acid to health and disease was drawn from various types of studies. These included observational, prospective, case control and intervention studies. Animal and laboratory data have also been considered to a limited extent. All types of studies have both advantages and disadvantages. Observational studies identify associations that are not necessarily causative. They are subject to various forms of bias, but can provide population-based estimates of the magnitude of the risk of disease associated with specific factors. Intervention studies (trials) can demonstrate causation, but care has to be taken in generalising their results beyond the particular subjects and circumstances involved. Judgement is required in combining data from the various types of study to provide an integrated picture.

2. Metabolism of folates and folic acid

2.1 Folate nomenclature

2.1.1 Folate is a generic term for compounds that have a common vitamin activity and includes the synthetic form of the vitamin folic acid (pteroyl glutamic acid) and a wide variety of derivatives. In this report we use the following terms:

(1) Folate/s: folic acid and its derivatives with the same vitamin activity;

(2) Folic acid (pteroyl glutamic acid): the core molecule; heat-stable, synthetic, not present in nature;

(3) Natural folate/s: natural compounds in foods that have the same vitamin activity as folic acid.

2.1.2 *Units of folate consumption* Folate intake is usually expressed in milligrams (mg) or micrograms (μg) per day. 1 g contains 1000 mg and 1 mg contains 1000 μg. In this report we use μg for values less than 1 mg and mg for values of 1 mg or greater. Folates in blood (serum and red blood cells) are usually expressed as nanomoles (nmol/l); 1 μg of folate represents 2.265 nmol.

2.2 Natural folate

2.2.1 Folate compounds all consist of the same basic structure that forms folic acid, an aromatic pteridine ring joined to p-aminobenzoate (to form a pteroyl moiety) and at least one glutamic acid residue (Figure 2.1). Natural folates differ from folic acid (pteroyl glutamic acid) in the following ways:

(1) They are reduced to di- or tetrahydroforms in the pteridine ring;

(2) They usually have additional single carbon units, e.g. methyl, methylene, methenyl, formyl;

(3) The main intracellular forms contain additional glutamate moieties, usually 4-6 linked by gamma-peptide bonds (folate polyglutamates). Folate polyglutamates are required as coenzymes in many reactions in 1-carbon unit transfer (Figure 2.2).

2.2.2 Dietary folates are absorbed through the duodenum and jejunum, where an enzyme, folate conjugase, in the mucosal brush borders and lysosomes of the enterocytes breaks down folate polyglutamates to monoglutamates. They are

15

also converted in the enterocytes to a single monoglutamate form, 5-methyl-tetrahydrofolate (5-methyl-THF). This is the form of folate generally present in plasma and other body fluids. 5-Methyl-THF passes from plasma into all body cells by diffusion. The folate monoglutamate 5-methyl-THF is not retained intracellularly unless it is metabolised by the vitamin B_{12}-dependent enzyme methionine synthase to tetrahydrofolate (THF) (Figure 2.2). This is because THF but not 5-methyl-THF can be conjugated into polyglutamate forms, thus preventing exit from the cell. If large doses of folic acid are consumed, and if the above mechanisms are saturated, free folic acid appears in the plasma.

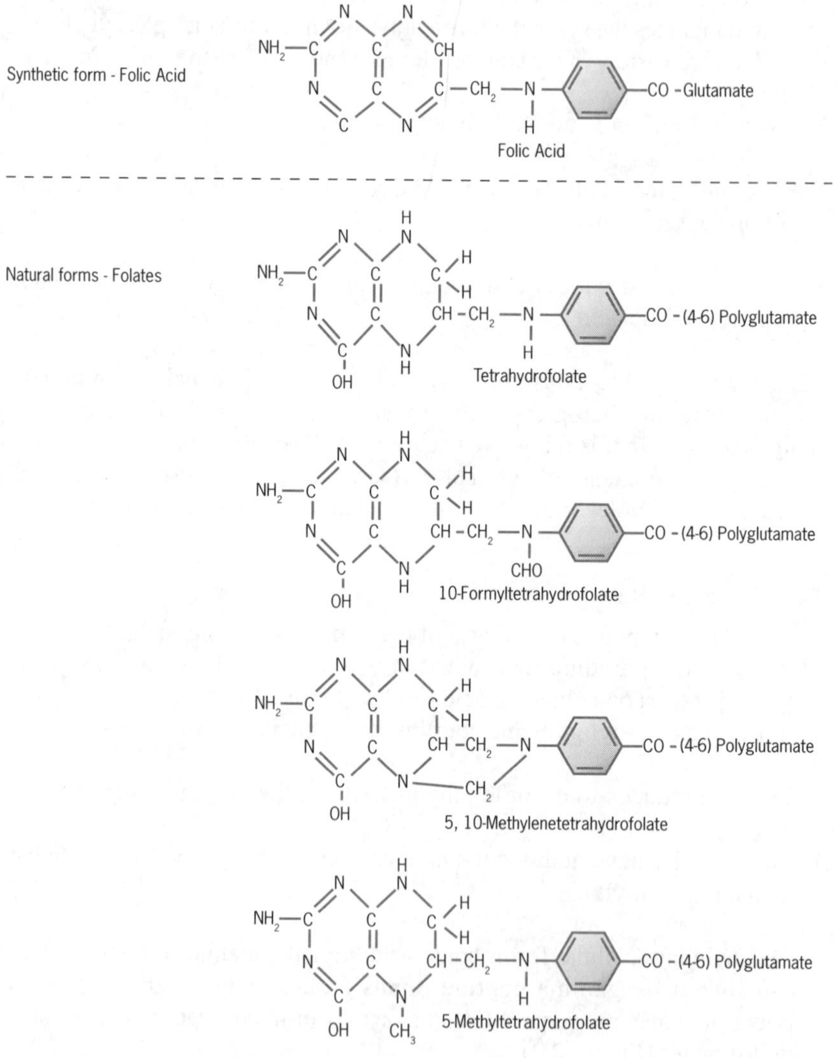

Figure 2.1. Formula of folic acid and tetrahydrofolic acid

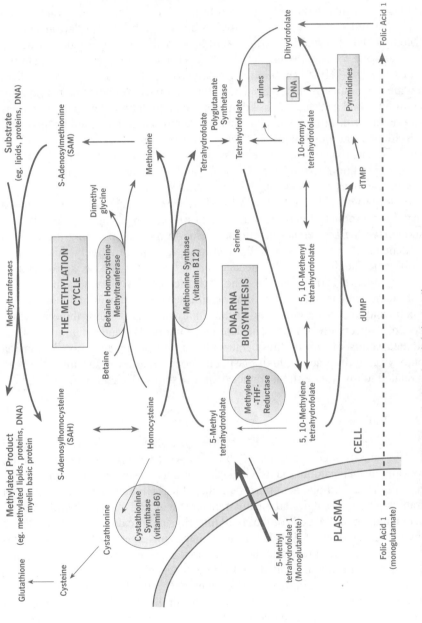

Figure 2.2. The role of folates in DNA biosynthesis and methylation reactions

Source: Scott and Weir (1998)[11]

2.2.3   The one-carbon units that are attached to intracellular folate include formyl, methylene and methenyl methyl groups (Figure 2.1); they are derived from serine and also probably from formate. They are used in the biosynthesis of pyrimidines and purines, and thus for the synthesis of DNA in cell division (Figure 2.2). As well as being essential for the action of the enzyme thymidylate synthase, and thus having a crucial role in DNA synthesis, 5,10-methylene-THF also indirectly supplies methyl groups for the "methylation cycle". 5-Methyl-THF is formed by reduction of 5,10-methylene-THF under the action of the enzyme 5,10-methylene-THF reductase. The methyl group is transferred from 5-methyl-THF to methionine, catalysed by the vitamin B_{12}-dependent enzyme methionine synthase. S-adenosylmethionine (SAM) is synthesised from methionine, and acts as a methyl donor in the methylation of a range of diverse compounds with different functions. The methyltransferase reactions give rise to S-adenosylhomocysteine (SAH), which is immediately metabolised to homocysteine. Excess homocysteine is usually broken down by the B_6-dependent enzyme cystathionine synthase to cysteine and pyruvate, which can be used for energy. Homocysteine may also be remethylated to methionine and hence used once more to provide the cell with SAM. Liver and kidney can use betaine, a breakdown product of choline independent of vitamin B_{12} and folate. All cells can achieve the conversion of homocysteine to methionine using the vitamin B_{12}-dependent enzyme methionine synthase, and quantitatively this is more significant. The 5-methyl-THF needed for methionine synthase is provided by 5,10-methylene-THF reductase. The activities of this enzyme and those of methionine synthase and cystathionine synthase keep the levels of homocysteine in cells and in plasma normally within a narrow range. These three enzymes depend, respectively, on folate, folate and vitamin B_{12} and vitamin B_6. Thus reduced status of any of these nutrients can cause an elevation in plasma homocysteine. In practice, high plasma homocysteine levels are most likely to be related to low folate status, rather than low status of vitamins B_6 or B_{12} [12].

2.3   Folic acid

Folic acid (pteroyl glutamic acid) itself is more stable chemically than natural folates, and it is not conjugated, both of which properties make it more bioavailable than natural folates when taken orally as a supplement or in fortified food (Figure 2.1). Folic acid must be reduced to THF and methylated before it acquires activity in single carbon unit transfer (Figure 2.2). This reduction usually occurs in the mucosal cells of the small intestine and is catalysed by the enzyme dihydrofolate reductase. This is followed by the conversion of THF to 5-methyl-THF, the usual form present in the circulation. The capacity for this conversion by the small intestine is limited, and single doses of folic acid that exceed 200 µg are not metabolised immediately, so that unaltered folic acid circulates in the plasma [13]. In that event, this folic acid is metabolised to THF inside the cells (including those of the bone marrow) or is excreted in the urine. Thus excess of folic acid intake results in body cells being presented with unaltered folic acid rather than 5-methyl-THF.

2.4   Effects of deficiencies

2.4.1   *Folate deficiency*   Folate deficiency affects rapidly dividing cells, particularly those of the bone marrow, causing megaloblastic erythropoiesis, macrocytosis of red cells and anaemia. There is commonly stomatitis and glossitis. It is rare for folate deficiency, on its own, to cause a neuropathy, although cases have been reported[14]. Folate deficiency has also been associated with a variety of neuropsychiatric disorders (Chapter 7). The folate level in cerebrospinal fluid is three times higher than that in plasma, and nerve tissue concentrates folate at the expense of other organs. This may account for the apparent protection of neural tissue from folate deficiency. Low folate status, even when serum and red blood cell folate levels are in the conventional normal range, is associated with an increased risk of neural tube defects. The levels required to prevent these defects are in excess of current estimates of folate requirements (Chapter 5), which may have implications for dietary reference values (Section 3.9). Low dietary intakes of folate (para 2.2.3) lead to raised homocysteine levels in plasma. A high level of homocysteine has been identified as a possible independent risk factor for occlusive vascular disease. Homocysteine can have a direct toxic effect on the vascular intima (Section 6.2).

2.4.2   *Vitamin B_{12} deficiency*   Vitamin B_{12} is required for activity of the enzyme methionine synthase, which enables the donation of a methyl group from 5-methyl-THF to homocysteine to form methionine and SAM. Deficiency of vitamin B_{12} is usually due to pernicious anaemia, in which there is inadequate absorption of vitamin B_{12} from the gastrointestinal tract because an autoimmune atrophic gastritis leads to the stomach failing to secrete the essential glycoprotein intrinsic factor needed for absorption of vitamin B_{12} through the ileum. Other gastric or small intestinal diseases may also cause deficiency. A vegan or vegetarian diet, which excludes animal products, may also lead to vitamin B_{12} deficiency, but this is rarely severe because the entero-hepatic circulation for vitamin B_{12} is intact. The clinical presentation is usually with megaloblastic anaemia or, in a smaller number of patients, with a neuropathy that may affect the spinal cord and the peripheral nerves (Section 7.2).

2.4.3   The metabolism of folate and vitamin B_{12} are linked. The enzyme methionine synthase, which is vitamin B_{12}-dependent, is essential for the conversion of 5-methyl-THF to THF. Only THF can act as substrate for synthesis of folate polyglutamates inside cells. In vitamin B_{12} deficiency, red cell folate is lower because lack of THF leads to failure of folate polyglutamate synthesis. Circulating plasma folate is higher than normal[15,16] presumably because of inability of red cells and other tissues to retain it. Folic acid, provided it is given in large enough doses, circulates free in plasma, enters cells and can then be metabolised into polyglutamates, including 5,10-methylene-THF polyglutamates, by mechanisms that are not vitamin B_{12}-dependent. This may explain the improvement in megaloblastic anaemia of vitamin B_{12} deficiency, in response to high doses of folic acid (e.g. 5 mg-13 mg daily). If anaemia caused by vitamin B_{12} deficiency improves with folic acid therapy, diagnosis could be delayed and the patient may present with the symptoms of neuropathy rather than those of anaemia. This is because the neuropathy is due to the interruption of the methylation cycle caused by reduced activity of vitamin B_{12}-dependent enzyme, methionine synthase. Folic acid, even after being metabolised to THF and 5-methyl-THF cannot restart this cycle (Figure 2.2).

2.4.4   In anaemia due to vitamin B_{12} deficiency, daily doses of folic acid between 1 and 5 mg produce a clear reticulocyte response (which indicates increased red cell production) and correction of anaemia[17]. Lower daily doses of folic acid are less likely to correct the anaemia of vitamin B_{12} deficiency. Doses of folic acid lower than 400 µg usually do not cause reticulocytosis in vitamin B_{12}-deficient anaemia, although there is some evidence that it might occur[17]. These considerations have led the US to introduce a national folic acid fortification policy, with the aim that folic acid intake should not exceed 1 mg daily.

2.4.5   Other functional markers have been identified for the early detection of vitamin B_{12} deficiency and to discriminate between deficiencies of vitamin B_{12} and folate. Both vitamins interact in the synthesis of methionine, and a deficiency of either is associated with elevated serum levels of the precursor homocysteine[18]. Under these conditions, increased urinary excretion of methylmalonic acid distinguishes vitamin B_{12} deficiency, which is specifically required for the conversion of methylmalonyl CoA to succinyl CoA.

2.5   Genetic aspects

A partial reduction of activity of 5,10 methylene tetrahydrofolate reductase (MTHFR) is a recognised genetic variant inherited in an autosomal recessive manner. This enzyme is involved indirectly in vitamin B_{12}-dependent remethylation of homocysteine to methionine in that it provides the 5-methyl-THF necessary for this remethylation (Figure 2.2). It is common, and homozygosity occurs in around 5-10% of the population. However, the frequency of homozygosity varies between populations; it was found in 38% of French Canadians and 5-15% of the general population in Canada[19,20]. The gene has been identified and is located on the short arm of chromosome 1. The phenotype is associated with three characteristics of low folate status, namely raised plasma homocysteine levels, increased risk of neural tube defects and increased risk of ischaemic heart disease. Homozygotes with this mutation also appear to have an exaggerated hyperhomocysteinaemic response to folate depletion and may be at higher risk of vascular disease[21]. Other inherited enzyme defects that may be relevant include cystathionine ß-synthase deficiency, a vitamin B_6-dependent enzyme involved in the conversion of homocysteine to cysteine (para 6.1.1) and methionine synthase deficiency, a vitamin B_{12}-dependent enzyme involved in remethylation of homocysteine to methionine. It is not known to what extent these genetic variants contribute to the detrimental effects of low folate intakes in the general population.

3. Dietary and nutritional aspects

3.1 Dietary Reference Values

3.1.1 Dietary Reference Values (DRV) for energy and nutrients were reassessed and set for the UK in 1991[22]. They define the estimated range of dietary requirements in different groups of individuals. They take account of the normal biological variation between individuals so that normal metabolic needs for healthy individuals, such as the requirements for growth, are taken into account. However DRVs make no allowance for the different energy and nutrient needs imposed by diseases.

3.1.2 For most nutrients, including folate, the DRVs comprise three levels of intake: the Estimated Average Requirement (EAR) of a group; the Reference Nutrient Intake (RNI), which is sufficient to cover the needs of nearly all the population group; and the Lower Reference Nutrient Intake (LRNI), sufficient only for those with the lowest requirements and unlikely to meet the needs of the majority. In developing these values, it is generally assumed that the distribution of requirements in the population for a nutrient is normal. On this basis, the RNI represents 2 notional standard deviations above, and the LRNI 2 notional standard deviations below the EAR, i.e. about 2.5% of the population will have requirements above the RNI, and 2.5% below the LRNI. Even when the distribution of intakes in a population is constant, the individuals representing the extremes are likely to vary from day to day.

3.1.3 Even if the distribution of intakes in a group of individuals is identical to that of their requirements for a nutrient, it is still probable that some individuals with lower intakes will have higher requirements, and *vice versa*. If there is no correlation between intakes and requirements in a group, then the average intake, even if equal to the EAR, carries a substantial risk of deficiency in the group represented by the upper dotted line in Figure 3.1, depicting risk. In order to avoid this risk completely, the distribution of intakes of the group would have to be such that the lowest intakes exceeded the highest requirements. If there is some correlation between intakes and requirements, then the greater that correlation the lower the risk. Body size may influence the relationships between intake and requirements, which in part determines energy requirements and therefore energy (and food) intakes. The degree to which this occurs is not known. The lower dotted line in Figure 3.1 takes account of this and represents the assessment of the actual risk of deficiency in a group. Furthermore, apparent requirements of individuals based on prevailing intake levels may not represent basal requirements. If an individual's intake falls below his/her usual intake, there may be adaptive mechanisms that reduce the risk of deficiency, which may not be fully evident until a period of time has elapsed, and this effect can vary for different nutrients. Adaptive mechanisms to handle nutrients consumed

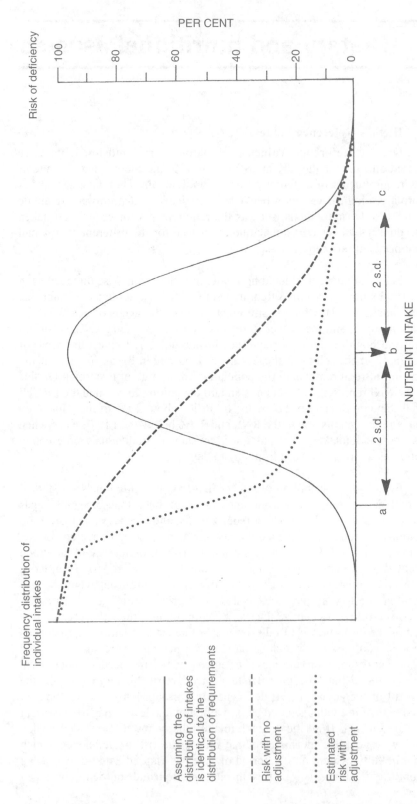

Figure 3.1 Dietary intakes and risk of deficiency

PER CENT

Risk of deficiency

100
80
60
40
20
0

Frequency distribution of individual intakes

NUTRIENT INTAKE

2 s.d.

2 s.d.

a

b

c

Assuming the distribution of intakes is identical to the distribution of requirements

Risk with no adjustment

Estimated risk with adjustment

in excess of requirements are not present for all nutrients. Excess amounts of fat-soluble vitamins (vitamins A and D), in particular, cannot be excreted, and high amounts have been shown to be toxic.

3.1.4   In the UK, a value for the Recommended Daily Amount (equates to current RNI) was set for folate for the first time in 1979, at 300 μg for adults[23]. Subsequently, the values for folate were withdrawn because of scientific uncertainties, particularly relating to the problems of biochemical assay of the active forms of this vitamin. In 1991, new values were declared based on balance studies which sought to titrate dietary intakes of folate against markers of folate status such as serum and red blood cell folate levels and the concentration of folate in the liver at post-mortem examination. The role of folate in the prevention of neural tube defects or as a determinant of plasma homocysteine was not used as a marker of status. The values for infants took account of the folate content of breastmilk. In the absence of scientific data, folate values for children were interpolated between the values for infants and those for adults. Increments were added during pregnancy and lactation to take account of the clinically recognised need for additional folate during later pregnancy to prevent megaloblastic anaemia, and for the replacement of folate secreted in breastmilk. The DRVs for folate are shown in Table 3.1.

Table 3.1   Dietary Reference Values for folate (μg/d)

Age	Lower Reference Nutrient Intake	Estimated Average Requirement	Reference Nutrient Intake
0-12 mth	30	40	50
1-3 yr	35	50	70
4-6 yr	50	75	100
7-10 yr	75	110	150
11 yr onwards	100	150	200
Pregnancy			+100
Lactation			+ 60

3.1.5   The European Union Scientific Committee for Food (SCF) set reference nutrient and energy intakes for adults in the European Union[24]. Those for folate requirements for adults vary a little from the UK values:

Lowest Threshold Intake (LRNI in UK) = 85 μg

Average Dietary Requirement (EAR in UK) = 140 μg

Population Reference Intake (RNI in UK) = 200 μg

23

3.1.6   The US National Academy of Sciences has recently published draft Reference Dietary Intakes, including revised Recommended Daily Allowance (RDA) for folate[25]. RDAs were estimated based on red cell folate as the primary indicator of folate status in conjunction with plasma homocysteine and folate concentrations. The revised RDA takes account of varying bioavailability of food folate and folic acid and is defined as Dietary Folate Equivalents (DFE). It is estimated that folic acid in food is 1.7 times more available than food folate, i.e.

Total folate intake (μg DFE) = μg of food folate + (1.7 $*$ μg of folic acid).

The RDA for all adults aged 19 years and over is 400 μg DFE/day.

3.1.7   In Great Britain, the Food Labelling Regulations 1996 (SI No 1499), implement European Community legislation on food labelling[26], and also sets out EC requirements on nutrition labelling[27], which specify the format, content and conditions of use for nutrition labelling. This includes recommended daily amounts (RDAs) for the purposes of making declarations for vitamins and minerals in nutrition labelling as a percentage of RDA. Similar but separate legislation exists for Northern Ireland. The RDA for folate (referred to as folacin) is 200 μg. Since the Directive has been in force, the SCF has been asked to advise on a set of nutrient values that should be used for nutrition labelling purposes. In its report, the SCF recommended a labelling reference value for folate of 140 μg/d, which is the estimated Average Dietary Requirement for adults. The nutrition labelling Directive is currently under review.

3.2   Food sources of folate

3.2.1   Folate was originally identified in green leafy vegetables and rich sources (>100 μg/serving) of this vitamin are Brussels sprouts, asparagus, spinach and kale. Other vegetables and fruits that contain lower but significant amounts (50-100 μg/serving) include broccoli, spring greens, cabbage, cauliflower, iceberg lettuce, parsnips and oranges[3]. Folate is concentrated in the liver, and this is a rich food source. It is also present in yeast, in yeast extract and in beer. In the British diet, the main sources of folate are cereals and vegetables (including potatoes), each contributing about a third of total folate intake. A significant proportion of the folate from cereals is derived from fortification, especially of breakfast cereals (Table 3.2).

3.3   Bioavailability of food folates and folic acid

The bioavailability of food folate is about 50% lower than that of folic acid[29]. It has been reported that natural folate resulted in a significantly smaller increase in red blood cell (RBC) folate concentration relative to folic acid supplements or folic acid in fortified cereals[30]. The absorption of stable-isotope labelled folic acid in cereal grain products was found to be approximately 15% lower than that when consumed with water[31]. Based on these data, the US Institute of Medicine, while acknowledging the imprecision of the calculation, estimated a bioavailability of 85% for folic acid from fortified foods, and that it is 1.7 times more bioavailable than food folate. In order to account for differences in

24

bioavailability of folates, the use of Dietary Folate Equivalents, on a similar basis to those used for other nutrients such as niacin, retinol or tocopherol, has been adopted by the US[25]. However, more studies are needed to characterise accurately the bioavailability and stability of folate in foods, particularly with regard to analytical methodology (Annex 3).

Table 3.2 Contribution of food groups to total folate content per head (natural folate and folic acid) of the household food supply in Great Britain for 1998[28]

Food group	Total folate/day	
	µg	% of total
Milk and milk products	24	9.8
- whole milk	7	2.9
- other milk and cream	12	4.9
- cheese	5	2.0
Total meat	13	5.3
Fish	3	1.2
Eggs	6	2.4
Fats	-	-
Sugars and preserves	-	-
Vegetables	78	31.8
- potatoes	25	10.2
- fresh green vegetables	19	7.8
- other fresh vegetables	15	6.1
- other vegetables and vegetable products	20	8.2
Fruit	17	6.9
Cereals	78	31.8
- bread	28	11.4
- breakfast cereals	35	14.3
Beverages	11	4.5
- tea	10	4.1
Other foods	9	3.7
TOTAL FOOD	**241**	**98.4**
Soft drinks	2	0.8
Confectionery	1	0.4
Alcoholic drinks	1	0.4
TOTAL FOOD AND DRINK	**245***	**100**

* Food and drink purchased and consumed outside the home contributed a further 29 µg/day in 1998.

3.4　Total folate (natural folate and folic acid) intakes in the UK

3.4.1　The average total folate intake per head of population in Britain in 1998 was 241 µg per day[28] (excluding soft and alcoholic drinks, confectionery, dietary supplements and food consumed outside the home). This is based on the results of the National Food Survey, which collects data on the amounts and costs of foods obtained by private households in Britain over a period of seven days. This survey gives information about long-term trends and showed that average intakes rose between 1980 and 1989, since when they have been relatively stable, with a relatively lower mean intake in Scotland than in England and Wales (Table 3.3). This trend can probably be ascribed to increasing fortification of breakfast cereals and to an increasing consumption of fruit and fruit juice. For example, in 1988, breakfast cereals contributed 6.5 µg/day to the folate intake, but by 1998 they contributed 35 µg/day owing to the introduction of fortification in these products. It is important to acknowledge that reliable determination of folate levels in foods is difficult and no present-day method is entirely satisfactory (Annex 3). This will inevitably have affected estimates of intake, particularly during the early 1980s. Folate is particularly sensitive to heat, and heating food in a neutral or alkaline media destroys folate. Methods of food preparation, such as canning, prolonged heating, discarding cooking water and reheating, can all cause serious losses of folate. The presence of reducing agents, such as vitamin C, can protect it from degradation.

3.4.2　Nationally representative data about the intakes of specific population groups are available from the National Diet and Nutrition Surveys, and other limited sources (Table 3.4). The most recent national data for adults aged 16-64 years are from 1986/87[32]; the information on the supplement use of 16-64 year olds therefore predates the various education campaigns on folic acid. Average intakes of folate in all age groups were above the RNI (200 µg/day), and less than 1% of men and 4% of women had intakes below the LRNI. Among adult women aged 16-64 years, 46% had folate intakes below the RNI[33]. For adults aged 65 years and over, mean intakes in all age groups for men and women, except women 85 years and over, were above the RNI, with men exceeding the RNI more than women[11]. A proportion of women had intakes from food sources below the LRNI of 100 µg; non-institutionalised older people – 4% at 65-74 years, 7% at 75-84 years, 11% at 85+ years; institutionalised older people – 2% at 65-84 years and 8% at 85+ years. Use of supplements made only a small difference to this proportion (Table 3.4). Fewer men had intakes below the LRNI. In the recent survey of 4-18 year olds, average folate intakes were above the RNI for boys and girls in all age groups. Three per cent of girls aged 11-14 years and 4% of girls aged 15-18 years had intakes below the LRNI[34]. Mean intakes for infants aged 6-12 months were approximately twice the RNI, and intakes at the 2.5 percentile were above the RNI[35]. Data from the NDNS of children aged 1½-4½ years show that mean intakes are well above the RNI for all age groups[10]. In all the surveys, the mean folate/folic acid intakes of subjects from manual households were lower than the mean intakes of those from non-manual households (Table 3.5).

Table 3.3 Total folate (natural folate and folic acid) content of the British household food supply 1980-1998[28]

Year	Total folate (µg/day)*			
	All households	England	Wales	Scotland
1980	213	214	222	197
1981	213	214	219	195
1982	208	210	207	184
1983	200	203	189	178
1984	200	203	197	176
1985	222	225	212	198
1986	231	232	239	215
1987	236	236	243	234
1988	230	230	223	228
1989	244	245	237	242
1990	244	243	246	247
1991	239	242	240	209
1992	243	244	244	230
1993	238	241	235	212
1994	238	241	243	208
1995	237	240	250	210
1996	248	250	243	234
1997	247	247	273	225
1998	241	242	258	223

* Excludes contributions from soft and alcoholic drinks and confectionery.

Table 3.4 Daily folate intakes (natural folate and folic acid) (μg) in Britain by age and sex

Age group & study	Year of fieldwork	Sex	Number studied	Mean Folate Intake (μg/day)		% Below the LRNI
				All sources (1SD)	Supplements	
6 – 9 months [35]	1986/7	Male	130	109 (27)	n/a	n/a
		Female	128	100 (26)	n/a	n/a
9 – 12 months[35]	1986/7	Male	96	111 (30)	n/a	n/a
		Female	134	104 (28)	n/a	n/a
1.5 – 2.5 years[10]	1992/3	Male	298	121 (43)	<1	0
		Female	278	120 (43)	<1	0
2.5 – 3.5 years[10]	1992/3	Male	300	136 (50)	<1	0
		Female	306	132 (50)	<1	0
3.5 – 4.5 years[10]	1992/3	Male	250	145 (50)	2	1
		Female	243	140 (49)	2	0
4 – 6 years[34]	1997/8	Male	184	192 (61)	1	0
		Female	172	171 (56)	2	0
7 – 10 years[34]	1997/8	Male	256	213 (61)	1	0
		Female	225	190 (57)	2	2
11 – 14 years[34]	1997/8	Male	237	247 (81)	2	1
		Female	238	210 (84)	5	3
15 – 18 years[34]	1997/8	Male	179	309 (124)	4	0
		Female	210	215 (82)	5	4
16 – 24 years [32]	1986/7	Male	214	302 (111)	<1	0
		Female	189	217 (234)	19	4
25 – 34 years[32]	1986/7	Male	254	319 (107)	2	0
		Female	253	208 (73)	2	6
35 – 49 years[32]	1986/7	Male	346	322 (105)	1	<1
		Female	385	224 (80)	4	2
50 – 64 years[32]	1986/7	Male	273	301 (97)	1	<1
		Female	283	222 (71)	4	2
65 – 74 years[11] *not institutionalised*	1994/5	Male	271	292 (110)	10	0
		Female	256	228 (95)	13	3
75 – 84 years[11] *not institutionalised*	1994/5	Male	265	256 (107)	7	1
		Female	217	217 (124)	16	6
65 – 84 years[11] *institutionalised*	1994/5	Male	128	234 (94)	0	4
		Female	91	211 (66)	1	1
85+ years[11] *not institutionalised*	1994/5	Male	96	242 (101)	8	4
		Female	170	192 (96)	8	11
85+ years[11] *institutionalised*	1994/5	Male	76	236 (95)	1	5
		Female	117	191 (68)	4	8

n/a = data not available   1 SD = one standard deviation

3.4.3   The Avon Longitudinal Study of Pregnancy and Childhood (ALSPAC) is a cohort study investigating factors influencing the health and development of infants and children[36]. Women with an expected delivery date between April 1991 and December 1992 were sent a self-completion questionnaire at 32 weeks' gestation. Dietary information was collected by means of food frequency questionnaire. Median estimated folate intake was below the RNI of 300 µg/day for early pregnancy (Table 3.6). Women who said that they had greater difficulty in affording food had lower folate intakes, probably because their consumption of green leafy vegetables, other green vegetables, salad, fruit and fruit juice was lower[37]. Nine per cent of women took folic acid supplements before 18 weeks' gestation and 18% at 32 weeks. However, advice from the Chief Medical Officer to all doctors on the use of folic acid in the prevention of neural tube defects was issued in August 1991[2].

3.4.4   A group of 963 nulliparous women, selected so that around a half of them were smokers, was recruited in south England between May 1994 and February 1996. Only 32% of women reported having taken supplements of folic acid prior to conception and 38% began taking folic acid supplements after conception[38]. Folate intake was assessed by a semi-quantitative 7-day food diary in 693 women between 14 and 17 weeks' gestation (early pregnancy) and in late pregnancy (28 weeks). Their median total folate intake was 261 µg/day in early pregnancy and 669 µg/day in late pregnancy. Folate intake from food in later pregnancy (28 weeks' gestation) was higher (median – 338 µg/day) as assessed by food frequency questionnaire[39] (Table 3.6).

Table 3.5   Mean total daily folate (natural folate and folic acid) intake from all sources (µg) by age, sex and social class of head of household

Age group & study	Year of fieldwork	Sex	Social class					
			I	II	IIINM	IIIM	IV	V
6 – 9 months[35]	1986/7	Both	104			105		
9 – 12 months[35]	1986/7	Both	104			108		
1½ – 4½ years[10]	1992/3	Both	134			130		
4 – 18 years*[34]	1997/8	Male	250			235		
		Female	200			188		
16 – 64 years[32]	1986/7	Male	321	298		317	294	
		Female	235	221		215	196	
65+ years[11] *Not institutionalised*	1994/5	Male	295			266		
		Female	239			209		

* these data are from food sources only

Table 3.6   Median total folate (natural folate and folic acid) intakes from food and supplements (µg/day) in pregnant women

Study	Number	Folate food sources only (µg/day)		Supplements (µg/day)
		Median	Range	
ALSPAC*[36]	11 923	245	138-378	n/a
Mathews**[39]	693			
Early		238	190-283	23
Late		338	279-421	331

* range = 5th percentile to 95th percentile   ** range = lower quartile to upper quartile

n/a = not available

3.5   Fortification of foods with folic acid

3.5.1   Fortification of foods with folic acid, as with other nutrients, is well established in the UK. Although folic acid is not naturally present in foods, it is readily absorbed and metabolised in the liver to the polyglutamate forms, which are indistinguishable from those derived from naturally occurring folates in food. Breads and breakfast cereals are the foods that have customarily been fortified with folic acid. There has been a rapid extension of the number of breakfast cereals available that are fortified with folic acid. It is estimated that between 80 and 90% of breakfast cereals consumed are fortified with folic acid. Muesli-type products, which are usually not fortified, make up around 11% of breakfast cereal consumption. Most folic acid fortified cereals claim to contain between 125 and 200 µg/100 g. Some products such as Kellogg's Cornflakes and Special K are fortified at a substantially higher level (333 µg/100 g). Fortification of bread is less widespread. The natural folate content of wholemeal bread is 37 µg/100 g. Most breads that are fortified claim to contain 118-120 µg folic acid/100 g. As part of the HEA Folic Acid Campaign, the availability of fortified breads was monitored (Annex 2). The number of types of loaf fortified with folic acid increased from 8 in December 1995 to 20 in December 1997[40], the majority being softgrain breads. Bread manufacturers have been reluctant to fortify a wider range of their products because of difficulties relating to labelling and the prohibition on making claims that a food may help prevent NTDs. There are also difficulties in providing alternative products within a high-turnover and mass-output industry with fierce price competition.

3.5.2   In the NDNS of 4-18 year olds, breakfast cereals, many of which are fortified, provided 25% of folate intake in males and 20% in females[34]. Tucker et al[41] examined the relationship between intake of food groups, specific sources of folate and plasma folate, and homocysteine concentrations in 885 elderly subjects in the Framingham Heart Study. Breakfast cereal consumers had significantly higher plasma folate and lower homocysteine levels than non-consumers.

3.6   Folic acid dietary supplements

3.6.1   Folic acid in doses of 500 µg or greater require medical prescription. Doses of 200-500 µg can be purchased at pharmacies over the counter, and lower doses are on general sale, but they may also all be prescribed where there is a medical need. The British National Formulary (BNF) notes that folic acid should not be prescribed alone in the presence of vitamin B_{12} deficiency "as it may precipitate the onset of subacute degeneration of the spinal cord"[42]. A common indication is the prevention or treatment of megaloblastic anaemia during the second half of pregnancy. Folic acid is also used to treat those at particular risk of folate deficiency because of clinical conditions such as malabsorption syndromes, coeliac disease, chronic alcoholism, chronic haemolytic states and those requiring renal dialysis. Folic acid supplements are advised for the prevention of neural tube defects (Annex 1). A dose of 5 mg daily is recommended to prevent recurrence of NTD where a previous child has been affected or in women with spina bifida themselves, and a dose of 400 µg daily to prevent first-time occurrence. The proportion of women claiming to take folic acid when planning for a baby rose from 24% in 1997 to 38% in 1998[40]. The 1995 Infant Feeding Survey[43] found that 75% of mothers knew that increasing their folic acid intake was good in early pregnancy. Mothers who had continued full-time education beyond the age of 16 and those in the higher social classes were more likely to say that they knew about the benefits of folic acid. Twenty six per cent of mothers had changed their diet and 50% had taken supplements; some had done both. These responses were collected retrospectively and therefore could have been influenced by current knowledge or a desire to give what they thought was the acceptable response. There are several preparations containing folic acid alone and others where folic acid is one of several micronutrients in the preparation. Sales of 400 µg folic acid supplements increased by 47% from the start of the HEA campaign in 1995. By autumn 1997, prescription rates for folic acid (400 µg) had increased by 55% from the start of the campaign.

3.6.2   The contribution of supplements to the folate intake of infants and pre-school children was found to be negligible[35,10], and for young people it was also small; supplements contributed less than 1% of total folate intakes for males aged 4 – 18 years and 1.5% for females[34]. In adults aged 16 – 64 years, vitamin supplements contributed little to total intake in 1986/87. Folate intakes were higher in supplement takers, even when the contribution from supplements was excluded. Supplements were more widely used in adults over 65 years not living in institutions contributing approximately 3% of total intake in men and around 6% in women[11].

3.7   Folate status

3.7.1   Representative data on the folate status of British population groups in this country are available from the three most recent National Diet and Nutrition Surveys. These cover children aged 1½ – 4½ years, young people aged 4 – 18 years and adults aged 65 years and over (Tables 3.7 and 3.8). The under-5s had satisfactory folate status as assessed by plasma or red blood cell folate levels. In the NDNS of 4 – 18 year olds, 1% of both males and females had serum folate levels lower than the reference value of 7 nmol/l (3.1 μg/l). Two per cent of young women aged 15 – 18 years had serum folate levels below this reference value and a significant proportion of this age group (10%) had red cell folate levels lower than the reference level of 345 nmol/l (152 μg/l).

3.7.2   A significant proportion of older adults (aged 65 years and over) had both serum folate and red blood cell folate in the range associated with tissue deficiency. The status was poorer in those living in institutions. The percentages falling below 7 nmol/l (3.1 μg/l) serum folate were 15% of those not in institutions and 39% of those in institutions. For red cell folate, 8% of those not living in institutions had levels below 230 nmol/l, indicating severe deficiency, whilst a further 21% had levels between 230 nmol/l and 345 nmol/l, indicating marginal status. In those living in institutions, 16% had levels below 230 nmol/l, whilst 19% had levels between 230 nmol/l and 345 nmol/l. Serum folate is a short-term indicator of status and so more reflective of recent variations in intake whereas red cell folate is more stable and reflects longer-term intake. The substantially lower mean serum folate levels in the institutionalised compared with those in the free-living groups is notable but not easy to explain as intakes of total folate between the groups were reported to be similar. This may reflect under-reporting by free-living individuals; or over-estimation of the food actually consumed by individuals living in institutions; or different proportions of the contribution from folic acid to total folate intake, as folic acid is more bioavailable. Inter-survey comparisons of folate status are complicated by the fact that different analytical methods have been used in different surveys (see Tables 3.7 and 3.8, and Annex 3).

Table 3.7 Mean plasma/serum folate* in British children aged 1½ – 4½ years, young people aged 4 – 18 years and adults aged 65+ years by age and sex (nmol/l and µg/l)

Age group & study	Year of fieldwork	Sex	Number Studied	Plasma/serum folate* nmol/l (1SD)	µg/l (1SD)**
1.5 – 2.5 years[10]	1992/3	Male	135	20.0 (9.3)	8.8 (4.1)
		Female	114	22.2 (10.2)	9.8 (4.5)
2.5 – 3.5 years[10]	1992/3	Male	165	20.6 (9.8)	9.1 (4.3)
		Female	152	21.5 (9.8)	9.5 (4.3)
3.5 – 4.5 years[10]	1992/3	Male	127	22.2 (10.2)	9.8 (4.5)
		Female	132	20.6 (8.8)	9.1 (3.9)
4 – 6 years[34]	1997/8	Male	85	25.0 (7.3)	11.0 (3.2)
		Female	82	25.8 (6.9)	11.4 (3.0)
7 – 10 years[34]	1997/8	Male	185	24.5 (6.9)	10.8 (3.0)
		Female	138	22.0 (8.5)	9.7 (3.8)
11 – 14 years[34]	1997/8	Male	181	20.8 (7.1)	9.2 (3.1)
		Female	168	19.3 (6.9)	8.5 (3.0)
15 – 18 years[34]	1997/8	Male	161	17.6 (7.0)	7.8 (3.1)
		Female	169	16.9 (7.5)	7.5 (3.3)
65 – 74 years[11] *not institutionalised*	1994/5	Male	212	15.2 (9.1)	6.7 (4.0)
		Female	192	16.8 (10.2)	7.4 (4.5)
75 – 84 years[11] *not institutionalised*	1994/5	Male	201	15.2 (10.7)	6.7 (4.7)
		Female	158	16.3 (10.9)	7.2 (4.8)
65 – 84 years *institutionalised*	1994/5	Male	89	9.5 (7.5)	4.2 (3.3)
		Female	59	12.2 (9.8)	5.4 (4.3)
85+ years[11] *not institutionalised*	1994/5	Male	69	17.0 (13.2)	7.5 (5.8)
		Female	112	17.2 (12.2)	7.6 (5.4)
85+ years[11] *institutionalised*	1994/5	Male	55	12.2 (10.7)	5.4 (4.7)
		Female	64	13.8 (12.0)	6.1 (5.3)

1 SD = one standard deviation

* Serum folate was measured by a radio-protein binding assay (BioRad Quantaphase I), an ion-capture assay (Abbot IMx) and a microbiological assay in the surveys of those aged 1½ – 4½, 4 – 18 and 65 years and over, respectively. For details, see individual reports of surveys (referenced above) and Annex 3.

** molecular weight of folic acid (441.4) used for conversion from SI units.

Table 3.8   Mean red blood cell folate* in British children aged 1½ – 4½ years, young people aged 4 – 18 years and adults aged 65+ years by age and sex (nmol/l and μg/l)

Age group & study	Year of fieldwork	Sex	Number studied	Red blood cell folate* nmol/l (1SD)	μg/l (1SD)**
1.5 – 2.5 years[10]	1992/3	Male	118	930 (383)	410 (169)
		Female	95	934 (333)	412 (147)
2.5 – 3.5 years[10]	1992/3	Male	300	930 (345)	410 (152)
		Female	306	837 (304)	369 (134)
3.5 – 4.5 years[10]	1992/3	Male	250	941 (306)	415 (135)
		Female	243	925 (340)	408 (150)
4 – 6 years[34]	1997/8	Male	79	736 (201)	325 (89)
		Female	77	677 (209)	299 (92)
7 – 10 years[34]	1997/8	Male	166	671 (199)	296 (88)
		Female	125	604 (223)	267 (98)
11 – 14 years[34]	1997/8	Male	172	598 (209)	264 (92)
		Female	163	544 (174)	240 (77)
15 – 18 years[34]	1997/8	Male	156	540 (181)	238 (80)
		Female	156	500 (171)	221 (76)
65 – 74 years[11] *not institutionalised*	1994/5	Male	212	494 (254)	218 (112)
		Female	180	481 (243)	212 (107)
75 – 84 years[11] *not institutionalised*	1994/5	Male	194	483 (306)	213 (135)
		Female	154	533 (340)	235 (150)
65 – 84 years *institutionalised*	1994/5	Male	83	415 (224)	183 (99)
		Female	59	499 (345)	220 (152)
85+ years[11] *not institutionalised*	1994/5	Male	69	562 (358)	248 (158)
		Female	110	510 (311)	225 (137)
85+ years[11] *institutionalised*	1994/5	Male	53	551 (474)	243 (209)
		Female	61	531 (345)	234 (152)

1 SD = one standard deviation

*   Red blood cell folate was measured by a radio-protein binding assay (BioRad Quantaphase I), an ion-capture assay (Abbott IMx) and a radio-protein binding assay (BioRad Quantaphase II) in the surveys of those aged 1½ – 4½, 4 – 18 and 65 years and over, respectively. For details, see individual reports of surveys (referenced above) and Annex 3.

** molecular weight of folic acid (441.4) used for conversion from SI units.

3.8 Folate status and plasma homocysteine concentrations

3.8.1 Plasma homocysteine levels are inversely associated with plasma and RBC folate levels (para 2.4.1). In the recent NDNS of adults aged 65 years and over, homocysteine levels were higher in individuals living in institutions, and there was a trend to increasing levels with age[44]. The dietary intakes of folate and vitamin B_6 were inversely related to the homocysteine levels (Table 3.9). Of the foods consumed, there were similar inverse relationships with the consumption of breakfast cereals (non-whole-grain, non-high-fibre) and of liver. There is also a trend to a poorer folate status in Scotland and the northern half of Britain (Table 3.10).

Table 3.9 Plasma total homocysteine in British adults aged 65 years or older (μmol/l)[44]

Domicile and age group	Sex	Number studied	Mean plasma homocysteine (μmol/l)
Not in institution			
65 – 74 years	Male	163	14.88
	Female	149	13.45
75 – 84 years	Male	151	17.12
	Female	136	15.69
85+ years	Male	61	18.16
	Female	88	17.43
All	Male	375	15.67
	Female	373	14.68
In institution			
65 – 74 years	Male	24	17.49
	Female	8	16.73
75 – 84 years	Male	47	20.07
	Female	38	21.00
85+ years	Male	50	20.11
	Female	57	21.58
All	Male	121	19.26
	Female	102	20.48
All participants	Male	496	16.21
	Female	476	16.18

Table 3.10 Regional variations in median plasma homocysteine, serum folate, red blood cell folate and serum B_{12} in those aged 65 years and over in Britain[44]

Region	Number studied	Plasma homocysteine (µmol/l)	Serum folate (nmol/l)	Red cell folate (nmol/l)	Serum B_{12} (pmol/l)
N England	125	15.7	10.2	391.2	198
Manchester/ Liverpool	95	15.0	12.2	407.9	229
S Midlands	167	15.7	11.8	403.2	201
E Anglia	83	14.1	13.6	441.5	215
London and SE	171	15.2	11.8	434.8	231
Central, South and South West	190	14.9	12.5	474.5	210
Wales	58	14.1	12.0	388.9	190
Scotland	83	16.7	10.0	366.5	191

3.8.2   Plasma homocysteine levels can be reduced by giving folic acid. A meta-analysis of randomised trials showed that folic acid supplements between about 1 mg and 5 mg reduce plasma homocysteine levels by about 25%[45]. The effect of folic acid in lowering homocysteine levels was greatest in the group with pre-treatment levels of homocysteine in the upper quintile of the distribution, but was also evident/significant in the group with lower pre-treatment levels of serum folate. The effect was similar with average doses between 500 µg and 5.7 mg folic acid, and in all groups the reduction of homocysteine levels amounted to about a quarter of the pre-treatment level. Where vitamin B_{12} had been added to the dose, there was an additional lowering of plasma homocysteine by about 7%.

3.8.3   A study of healthy men (mean age 45 years) measured the effect on plasma homocysteine concentrations of folic acid in daily doses of 100, 200 and 400 µg given for several weeks[46]. Homocysteine levels were lowered in the top and middle tertiles only. Of the three doses, 200 µg appeared to be as effective as 400 µg in lowering plasma homocysteine in apparently normal subjects, but 100 µg was clearly not optimal. In a placebo-controlled study[47], 144 healthy women aged 18 – 40 years were given 500 µg of folic acid/day or 500 µg every second day or a placebo for 4 weeks, with their habitual diet providing 280 µg/day of dietary folate. There was a significant decrease in plasma homocysteine concentration (–11.4% ± 1.98% in women who took 500 µg of folic acid every second day, and –21.8 ± 1.49% in women who took a daily dose of 500 µg of folic acid). The levels remained below that of baseline, 8 weeks after cessation of supplements.

3.8.4   In a randomised double-blind placebo-controlled crossover trial, men and women were given fortified breakfast cereals that provided 127 µg/day or 499 µg/day of folic acid for a period of 5 weeks. Additional intake of folic acid at different levels reduced plasma homocysteine levels by 3.7, 11 and 14%, respectively[48]. The effect of a small increase in folic acid in food on plasma homocysteine levels was studied in a randomised double-blind placebo-controlled trial by Schorah et al[49]. Healthy volunteers (n=94) with low intake of fortified or supplemental folic acid were randomised to receive unfortified cereals or cereals fortified with 200 µg/portion (666 µg/100 g) of folic acid, with or without other vitamins (B_1,B_2, niacin, B_6, B_{12}, C and D). Fasting blood samples were taken before intervention and after intervention at 4, 8 and 24 weeks and analysed for serum and red cell folate, vitamin B_{12}, homocysteine and cysteine. There were no significant changes in any of the measured parameters in those who consumed unfortified cereals. Overall folic acid intake of 200 µg/day led to a significant increase in serum folate (66% p<0.001) and red cell folate (24%). Plasma homocysteine levels decreased by 10% (p<0.001) and the decrease persisted throughout the duration of the study. The significant decrease was primarily seen in those who initially had the highest plasma homocysteine or lowest serum folate.

3.9   Review of the current DRV for folate

3.9.1   The current folate DRV is based on its requirement for the avoidance of megaloblastic anaemia, and red cell folate concentration is used as a marker of adequacy, contingent on its known relationship to blood haemoglobin levels. A variety of new data has accumulated since 1991 which needed consideration as to whether they provided an appropriate and/or sufficient base for a revision of the DRV. In particular, there is evidence that a modest daily increase in folic acid of around 100 µg to 200 µg/day can significantly reduce the risk of NTDs[50] and also lower plasma homocysteine levels[49].

3.9.2   As part of the programme of this Working Group, a meeting was held specifically to discuss whether there was a need to revise the current UK DRV for folate in the light of developing knowledge, and in particular whether a raised homocysteine could be used as the functional marker of folate deficiency. The Working Group concluded that folate status was an important determinant of blood levels of homocysteine, but that there were also a number of other dietary and non-dietary factors (Sections 2.2 and 2.3). In addition, there was considerable variation amongst the population in blood levels of homocysteine, and it was not certain how much of this was due to variations in folate status. There is also a lack of information on prevailing levels of homocysteine in healthy adults below 65 years of age. Furthermore, although evidence was accumulating on the different efficiencies of absorption and utilisation of various forms of folate (including folic acid), and of the genetic and other determinants of this, there was still considerable uncertainty about how to translate this practically into a revised DRV (for instance by the use of folate equivalents) (Section 3.3). In view of these remaining uncertainties, COMA accepted the recommendation of the Working Group that, although there was insufficient evidence to revise the DRV at the present time, the issue should be addressed as soon as practicable, and that this should form part of any more general review of DRVs for other nutrients, and of the philosophy underlying them.

4. Folate/folic acid and early pregnancy

4.1 Formation of the neural tube

4.1.1 The development of the brain and spinal cord becomes evident around day 18 after conception, with a localised thickening of cells known as the neural plate. This becomes elongated and a longitudinal fold from each side of this plate progressively overarches and finally fuses with its opposite in the midline. This neural tube closes first at the midbrain/cervical region about 21 days after conception, then at the cephalic end around day 24, and finally at the posterior end around day 26. The neural tube is destined to form the brain and spinal cord; eventually, the central neural canal becomes insignificant compared with the substantial growth of nervous tissue cells. The closed neural tube then induces development in the surrounding mesoderm to build up the bony structures destined to become the vertebral column and the skull. However, the bone fails to form above any unclosed region of the neural tube and this leads to the congenital malformations collectively known as neural tube defects. The site of the defect depends on the location along the neuraxis at which closure of the neural tube fails to occur. If the cephalic part of the tube is affected, the outcome is anencephaly, while if any of the remainder is affected, the outcome is spina bifida. Encephaloceles (which are rare compared with anencephaly and spina bifida) are small localised lesions in the head.

4.1.2 The nutrient needs of the embryo throughout the first 21-22 days are provided by diffusion through the cytotrophoblast from the uterine glands. Beyond this date, a heart beat is established and a circulation of fetal blood begins to distribute nutrients to the developing fetal tissues. Thus, during the critical period from day 21-22 to the closure of the neural tube, nutrients are provided both by diffusion and, increasingly, by the developing circulatory system. The developmental processes in the embryo occur rapidly and involve frequent cell division, and so demand an adequate and assured supply of nutrients. (A fuller description of these processes is at Annex 4.)

4.2 NTD in early spontaneous abortion

4.2.1 A high proportion of pregnancies ends in spontaneous abortion in the first trimester. In such abortuses, neural tube defects are found in 3-6% of recognisable embryos, which is a much higher frequency than is seen at birth. Most of these are likely to have arisen through causes other than folate status, chromosome abnormalities being the most common[51,52].

39

4.2.2   In the first trimester group, more than half of all neural tube defects are associated with chromosome abnormalities, 53% in one study[51] and 80% in another[52], while at birth, very few are associated with chromosome abnormalities. Further, the types of neural tube defects differ between the two groups. At term, anencephaly is common, with or without spina bifida (40% of NTDs), as is spina bifida (55%), while encephalocele is uncommon (5%). In the first trimester, encephaloceles are very common (42%) and a caudal hyperplasia and protrusion of the neural tissue, not seen in later pregnancy, is the next most common (34%). Classical spina bifida is found in only 18%, while anencephaly accounts for only 5%. All these observations suggest that the two populations of neural tube defects are constitutionally and aetiologically different. In the early embryos, there is no correlation between the particular chromosome abnormality and the type of neural tube defect. Encephalocele is found in trisomy, triploidy and X monosomy, as well as with normal chromosomes. Classical spina bifida and anencephaly are found in trisomy and triploidy, and with normal chromosomes. Further, there are no specifically associated forms of trisomy: NTDs have been observed in cases of trisomy 9, 13, 14, 15, 16, 18, 20 and 21 - generally all those where a recognisable embryo can develop. In these cases, neural tube defects may simply be a sign of disordered growth associated with aneuploidy in general.

4.3   Other congenital abnormalities

Other congenital abnormalities, such as facial clefts and harelip, have been linked to a relative lack of folate[53], but the evidence of a direct protective effect of folate remains uncertain[54].

4.4   Multiple births and terathanasia

It has been suggested that some agents that reduce the incidence of birth defects might do so by increasing the rate of death or abortion of affected fetuses ("terathanasia") and that the effect of folic acid on NTDs could be mediated by this means. For this reason, there has been some concern over an increased rate of spontaneous abortions among women taking folic acid supplements[55,56]. This is most likely due, however, to an increase in fertility and multiple pregnancies among women taking supplements and to an effect of folate in allowing the survival of non-viable conceptuses to a stage where their loss is recognised as abortions[57]. The generally accepted view is that folic acid supplements prevent NTDs simply by allowing the normal development of the fetal neural tube.

4.5   Birthweight

Folate supplementation during pregnancy may reduce the incidence of low-birthweight infants, but the reported studies are criticised as being of poor quality[58] and most have included supplementation with other vitamins and minerals. We found no data linking birthweight with preconception dietary fortification.

5. Folate/folic acid and the prevention of neural tube defects

5.1 Background

5.1.1 During the early 1960s, studies in Liverpool investigated the relationship between adverse outcome in pregnancy and vitamin status. The women were poor, many were born in Ireland, and many had very large families. The high rate of megaloblastic anaemia during pregnancy drew attention to the common condition of folate deficiency. Folate status was assessed by the formiminoglutamic acid excretion test (FIGlu), and other conventional haematological assessments, which included examining the bone marrow. An association was found between a positive FIGlu test, which was taken to denote folate deficiency, and central nervous system malformations of the fetus; in a group of infants thus affected, the FIGlu test was positive in 69%, while the FIGlu test was positive in only 17% of a matched group of infants with no such abnormalities[59]. Mindful of the tendency for these malformations to recur in affected families, the paper speculated that "The familial occurrence of serious nervous system malformations might be mediated, in some instances, through a genetically determined defect of folate metabolism."

5.1.2 In 1998, 93 children were notified as being born with NTD in the UK[60]. It is difficult to ascertain the numbers of affected pregnancies, but it has been estimated that, without screening and selective termination, there would have been about 600 – 1200 affected births[61,62]. There are variations in the prevalence of neural tube defect dependent on ethnic, demographic and social factors[63]. Rates are influenced by race; for example, high rates occur in people of Welsh, Irish and South Asian origin. However, migrants from an area with a high prevalence of NTD who move to an area with a low prevalence acquire a new lower risk, which indicates that environmental factors influence the risk. Within populations, women in poverty and women at the extremes of the reproductive period are at greater risk.

5.2 Folate levels in blood

5.2.1 An early study in Aberdeen found no relationship between serum folate levels in early pregnancy and risk of neural tube defect[64]. However, in 1976, the Leeds Pregnancy Nutrition Study reported a significant difference between the mean red blood cell folate level from 6 NTD pregnancies when compared with the mean from some 1000 pregnancies without NTD. The mean serum folate levels showed a similar trend between the two groups, with NTD pregnancies having a significantly poorer folate status[65]. Similar observations were reported from the west of Scotland[66], as well as from Dublin[67] but there were no differences in the mean levels of serum folate in comparative groups in Finland[68]. The Dublin study also found a significantly lower plasma vitamin B_{12} in the NTD pregnancies[69]. Further results from this group showed that the group of NTD mothers had a significantly higher mean level of homocysteine than the control group. The mean level of methylmalonic acid was similar in case and control groups. This further analysis suggested that the abnormality in the metabolic pathways might relate to the enzyme methionine synthase[70].

5.2.2   It has been suggested that the discrepancy between the results from different studies can be explained by a combination of factors. The numbers of cases in individual studies were small and the range of serum folate levels in the population studied was narrow, thereby minimising the ability of an individual study to demonstrate a dose-response relationship between blood folate indices and the risk of neural tube defects. This phenomenon has been described as the "narrow window effect". Meta-analysis of all the blood studies has confirmed the association between low blood folate and risk of neural tube defects[71].

5.3   Folate/folic acid intake and risk of NTD

5.3.1   These observations raised the question of whether risk of an NTD pregnancy might be reduced by improving the mother's folate status before conception. The first intervention study was reported from south Wales[72] and assessed the effect of dietary counselling to "improve their diet". The quality of diets of 174 women who had previously had a child with an NTD was assessed retrospectively during the first trimester of that pregnancy, between pregnancies and during the first trimester of other pregnancies. They were then studied prospectively during the first trimester of following pregnancies. One hundred and three women were given dietary counselling "to improve their diet", and the remaining 71 women were not counselled. There were three recurrences of NTDs in the counselled women compared with five in uncounselled women. Although the difference was not statistically significant, all eight affected pregnancies were in the group of 45 women in whom the quality of the diet was assessed to be poor. The results relating to the effectiveness of dietary counselling were found to be equivocal, which probably reflects the difficulty of persuading people to change their diet.

5.3.2   *Non-randomised intervention studies with dietary supplements*   Several intervention studies have improved folate status of the mother by supplementing the diet periconceptionally with folic acid either singly or as a part of a micronutrient supplement. An intervention trial in Cuba using 5 mg of folic acid supplementation, but with small numbers of participants, also showed a significant reduction in relative risk[73] (see Table 5.1). In an intervention study on a UK-wide population group, Pregnavite Forte F* was offered to women

---

* vitamin A 3 µg, vitamin D 10 µg, thiamin 1.5 mg, pyridoxine 1.5 mg, nicotinamide 15 mg, vitamin C 40 mg, folic acid 0.36 mg, ferrous sulphate equivalent to 75.6 mg of iron, calcium phosphate 480 mg

with a history of NTD pregnancy, to be taken not less than 28 days before conception through to the time of the second missed menstrual period. There was a significant reduction in NTD pregnancies: 1 out of 178 infants/fetuses of fully supplemented mothers, when compared with 13 out of 260 infants/fetuses of unsupplemented mothers[74]. Similar results were subsequently reported in regional studies[75,76]. The effectiveness of periconceptional vitamin supplementation for the prevention of recurrence of NTDs varied according to extremes of prevalence in different regions. Seller and Nevin[63,77] showed a differential effect in south east England compared with Northern Ireland, which had a higher prevalence. The rate of recurrence in south east England was more than twice that found in Northern Ireland, indicating that vitamin supplementation was effective in primary prevention of NTD where prevalence is high, but less so where prevalence is lower. Environmental (dietary) contribution to risk of NTD might be greater in high- than in low-incidence areas. A large trial in China, which included over 160,000 women from high-risk northern districts and low-risk southern districts, showed that daily periconceptional supplementation with 400 µg of folic acid significantly reduced the risk of NTDs. A reduction in risk of 79% (95% CI 57-90%) in the northern district and 41% (95% CI –19-80%) in the southern districts was observed[78].

Table 5.1   Use of vitamin supplements in non-randomised trials to prevent recurrence of NTD[79]

Study	Type of supplement	Folic acid (mg/day)	No. of pregnancies	No. of NTDs	Relative risk	95% CI
Smithells et al[80]	Multinutrient	0.36	973	27	0.14	0.03-0.47
Vergel et al[73]	Folic Acid	5	195	4	0.00	0.00-2.13
Combined	-	-	1168	31	0.12	0.04-0.41

5.3.3   *Randomised intervention studies with dietary supplements* Definitive evidence that supplementing with folic acid can prevent neural tube defects comes from the results of randomised controlled trials. Various reviews have been published[81,82]. Four trials have been carried out; these are summarised in Table 5.2. There were 40 pregnancies associated with neural tube defects in the four trials. The rate of neural tube defects in the supplemented women was 76% lower than in women receiving no supplements. Two of the trials used 4.0 mg of folic acid; one trial used 800 µg, and one used 360 µg, although this one was based on only one case of neural tube defect. The MRC Vitamin Study[1] tested the effect of other vitamins (vitamin A, B_2, B_6, C, D and nicotinamide), but these did not result in a statistically significant reduction in risk of NTDs.

Table 5.2 Use of vitamin supplements in randomised control led trials[79]

Trial	Recurrence (R) or occurrence (O)	Folic acid (FA) or multinutrient (M)	Daily dose of folic acid supplement (mg)	Number of pregnancies	Number of neural tube defects	Relative risk	95% Confidence interval
MRC Vitamin Study Research Group[1]	R	FA	4	1031	27	0.29	0.10-0.74
Laurence et al[83]	R	FA	4	111	6	0.42	0.04-2.97
Kirke et al[84]	R	FA	0.36	261	1	0.00	Insufficient data
Czeizel and Dudas[56]	O	M	0.8	4156	6	0.00	0.00-0.85
Combined	-	-	-	5559	40	0.24	0.11-0.52

5.3.4   Observational studies in the general population collectively show that women on folic acid supplements (either alone or together with other vitamins) have a lower risk of neural tube defect pregnancy than other women. These observations are important in assessing the effectiveness of folic acid in preventing first-time occurrence, because previous studies had included only participants with a history of a previous NTD. The results of these studies are summarised in Table 5.3. All the observational studies show a relative risk less than 1 (risk of neural tube defects in supplemented women less than in unsupplemented) and in four of these the differences were individually statistically significant.

Table 5.3   Observational studies of the use of vitamin supplements containing folic acid and prevention of first occurrence of NTD: dose of folic acid was about 400 µg/day[79] (modified from Wald[79])

Study	Relative Risk[a] (95% confidence interval)
Winship et al[85]	0.14 (0.003-1.11)
Mulinare et al[86]	0.41 (0.26-0.66)
Mills et al[b 87]	0.94 (0.80-1.10)
Milunksy et al[88]	0.29 (0.15-0.55)
Werler et al[89]	0.6 (0.4-0.9)
Bower & Stanley[c 90]	0.11 (0.01-1.33)
All studies combined	0.47 (0.29-0.76)

a   Relative risk estimate given is that cited by the authors and may be adjusted for possible confounding factors.

b   The relative risk cited was based on the use of normal controls; it was 0.87 (0.73-1.02) using controls with congenital abnormalities other than neural tube defects.

c   The relative risk was 0.69 (0.06-8.53) for controls with congenital abnormalities other than neural tube defects.

5.3.5   *Effective dose of folic acid*   Intervention studies using low doses of folic acid have been undertaken to assess the minimum dose of folic acid that will prevent NTD in the general population. In a randomised placebo-controlled trial Daly et al[50] assigned 121 women to receive placebo, 100 µg, 200 µg or 400 µg of additional folic acid daily and measured the resulting red cell folate levels, allowing the authors to estimate the likely change in risk of NTD. Subjects with red cell folate concentrations at screening within the range of 150 µg to 400 µg/l were included in the study. The estimated reduction in the risk of NTD was greater in those women whose red cell folate levels were <400 µg/l at the

45

start of the trial than in those whose levels were >400 µg/l at the start of treatment. There was a progressive decrease in the estimated risk of NTD with increasing dose of folic acid intake (22% for 100 µg, 41% for 200 µg and 47% for 400 µg). The authors concluded that supplementation with doses of folic acid in this range could have a significant impact on risk of NTDs in the general population. Based on the same data, Wald *et al* calculated reductions of 18%, 35% and 53%, respectively[91].

6. Homocysteine and vascular disease

6.1 Background

6.1.1 Homocysteine is a sulphur-containing amino acid (para 2.2.3). Total homocysteine (tHcy) is the sum of homocysteine plus homocysteinyl moieties of oxidised disulphides, homocystine and cysteine-homocysteine. Inborn errors of metabolism affecting the enzymes involved in homocysteine metabolism cause markedly elevated levels of homocysteine (para 2.2.3). Affected children suffer from early-onset occlusive vascular disease with the pathological features of atherosclerosis irrespective of the precise genetic disorder, with hyperhomocysteinaemia being the common factor. This observation has led to speculation that moderately elevated levels of homocysteine, or its derivatives, might contribute to vascular disease in the general population.

6.1.2 At least one, possibly more, genetic variants are associated with hyperhomocysteinaemia in otherwise normal adults. In northern European populations, there is a homozygote frequency of around 10% of a single base substitution in the gene controlling the production of the enzyme 5-methyl tetrahydrofolate reductase (MTHFR), which results in reduced activity of this enzyme. *In vitro*, it is more thermolabile than the usual form of the enzyme[92]. Individuals homozygous for this mutation tend to have raised plasma homocysteine levels more so in the presence of lower plasma folate levels, less so if folate is above the median[93]. Mean plasma homocysteine levels have been reported from 11 populations in Europe as well as Japan and Israel and compared with the local cardiovascular disease mortality rate. There were significant differences in the mean plasma homocysteine levels recorded for people from different countries, and diversity in the size of the standard deviations of the distributions. Although the reason for this diversity is not known, there was a positive relationship between plasma total homocysteine and cardiovascular mortality. It is possible that differences in the genetic profile of populations account in part, but dietary factors, especially folate intakes, may be implicated[94]. A number of studies have demonstrated that folic acid administration can lower plasma homocysteine. Breakfast cereal fortification with folic acid at a level of 127 µg/d had a small effect (decrease of 3.7%) on plasma homocysteine levels, but levels of 499 µg/d and 665 µg/d reduced homocysteine levels significantly, by 11% and 14% respectively[48]. The distribution of MTHFR genotypes was similar in the study groups and did not contribute to differences in the homocysteine lowering among the three groups.

6.1.3 Many studies have examined the relationship between plasma homocysteine and the risk of vascular disease in adults. Twenty-seven studies were examined in a meta-analysis published in 1995[7]. The majority of the study populations were middle-aged men. They included cross-sectional and prospective studies and population-based case control studies. Plasma homocysteine levels increased with age, and elevation of total homocysteine showed a linear graded association with risk of vascular disease in most, but not all, of the studies. Vascular disease at several sites has been examined, including coronary and carotid arteries[95], the cerebral vasculature[96], the peripheral arteries and arterial disease in lupus erythematosus, as well as deep-vein thrombosis[97]. There was agreement across the studies that, where an association was found, it was independent of other known risk factors for vascular occlusive disease, such as blood cholesterol, obesity and smoking. The meta-analysis estimated that, if plasma homocysteine levels were reduced by 5 µmol/l, the mortality from coronary artery disease would be reduced by about 10% in US men aged 45 and over 6% in women[7]. Since that time, there has been a large number of published reports of more recent observational studies (Section 6.3).

6.1.4   Since the publication of the 1995 meta-analysis cited in para 6.1.3, there have been several further epidemiological studies on the relationship between plasma homocysteine and CHD. A systematic review[98] included five nested case control studies involving a total of 1041 cases, with a weighted mean age at baseline of 53 years and a mean follow-up of 8 years. An increase in plasma homocysteine of 5 µmol/l was associated with a combined odds ratio of 1.3 (95% CI 1.1-1.5). The role of plasma homocysteine in the causation of CHD requires further study to determine the strength of the association and any dose-response relationship with risk, and take account of all potential confounding factors, particularly the within-individual variations in homocysteine levels over time.

6.1.5   Few studies have included older people (65 years or older). Normative values for plasma total homocysteine have recently been published for the British population aged 65 years and older[44] (para 3.8.1). The mean plasma homocysteine levels reported from the Framingham cohort (13.0 (SD 5) µmol/l for men and 12.5 (SD 6) µmol/l for women[96]), now aged about 75 years, were lower than comparable UK values (16.2 (SD 8) µmol/l in both men and women[44]).

6.2   **Possible mechanisms**

Experimental evidence suggests that the atherogenic propensity associated with raised homocysteine levels results from endothelial dysfunction and injury followed by platelet activation and thrombus formation. Plausible biological mechanisms have been proposed. Homocysteine has been shown to promote oxidative modification of LDL cholesterol, which can promote the formation of atherosclerotic lesions. It can also have a direct effect on vascular endothelium by stimulating the proliferation of vascular smooth muscle cells. Homocysteine can alter the normal antithrombotic mechanisms by enhancing the activities of factor XII and factor V and depressing the activation of protein C[99-101]. In addition, homocysteine reduces the production of endothelial-derived nitric oxide, which has vasodilatory effects. Normal endothelial cells detoxify homocysteine by releasing nitric oxide, which combines with homocysteine in the presence of oxygen to form S-nitroso-homocysteine, a potent platelet inhibitor and a vasodilator. The protective effect of nitric oxide is eventually compromised, as long-term exposure to raised homocysteine levels damages the endothelium sufficiently to limit the production of nitric oxide. Impaired endothelium-dependent vasodilation and endothelial anticoagulant function have been found in young patients with hyperhomocysteinaemia and peripheral vascular disease[102,103].

6.3   Results of studies in populations from the UK

6.3.1   The British Regional Heart Study examined prospectively the relationship of serum homocysteine levels to risk of stroke. This was a nested case control study of 5661 middle-aged men living in 24 towns throughout Britain. Serum samples were taken between 1978 and 1980. Twelve years later, 141 cases of stroke, both fatal and non-fatal, had been verified. The mean level of homocysteine (13.7 µmol/l) was significantly higher in the cases (107 men) when compared with the 118 matched controls selected for this study (mean 11.9 µmol/l). The odds ratio as a measure of relative risk of stroke, between the lowest and the highest quartiles of homocysteine level, was 4.1 (95% CI 1.6-10.5). This relationship was unchanged after adjusting for known risk factors for stroke, such as blood pressure, body mass index and serum cholesterol and creatinine concentrations[104].

6.3.2   The British United Provident Association[8] study examined prospectively the relationship of homocysteine levels to risk of coronary heart disease in a nested case control study of 229 men who had died from ischaemic heart disease, and 1126 matched controls. Serum samples were taken and stored between 1975 and 1982 from men aged 35-64 years. All the cases had been free of evidence of coronary heart disease at recruitment and had subsequently died of the disease. The mean homocysteine concentration in the coronary heart disease group was 13.1 µmol/l compared with 11.8 µmol/l in the matched controls, and ranged from 5.9 to 52.2 µmol/l and 4.3 to 44.9 µmol/l, respectively. The relative risk between the lowest and the highest quartile was 2.9 after adjustment for apolipoprotein B and systolic blood pressure (95% CI 1.79-4.68). Serum homocysteine was correlated with systolic blood pressure and levels of serum apolipoprotein B, but not with serum apolipoprotein A_1 or with smoking[8]. This study concluded that a reduction of plasma homocysteine of 0.9 µmol/l was associated with a 10% decrease in risk of occlusive vascular disease (95% CI 4-16%).

6.3.3   A separate multicentre study in Northern Ireland and France quotes homocysteine levels for Belfast men and men from Lille and Strasbourg; data from the last two locations are combined as France[105]. This was an observational study using the cohort from the World Health Organization MONICA (multinational monitoring of trends and determinants in cardiovascular disease) project. The mean plasma homocysteine level of 171 Belfast men aged 25-64 years without myocardial infarction was 14.7 µmol/l, and of 191 survivors of myocardial infarction was 15.5 µmol/l. This compared with a mean plasma homocysteine level of 12.9 µmol/l in 315 French controls and 16.7 µmol/l in 229 French survivors of myocardial infarction. After adjustment for confounding factors, log homocysteine levels did not differ significantly between cases and controls in Belfast. There was a graded risk when the homocysteine levels were divided as deciles, but this lost statistical significance when a wide range of risk factors for myocardial infarction were introduced into the analysis. In comparison with the results from the study participants in France, the generally higher homocysteine levels of the controls in Belfast is notable. The paper suggests that the threefold higher rate of myocardial infarction in Northern Ireland, when compared with France, might, in part, be due to higher plasma homocysteine levels in the population as a whole.

6.3.4   South Asians living in the UK are known to have a higher prevalence of diabetes and heart disease than the white population. Plasma homocysteine concentrations were measured in 170 South Asians (Bangladeshis) in East London[106]. Fasting blood samples were obtained and 75.4% were found to be normoglycaemic, 16.4% had impaired glucose tolerance, and 8.2% were diagnosed as diabetics. Mean homocysteine level in plasma was 13.3 µmol/l (range: 5.7 to 42 µmol/l). A large proportion had raised homocysteine levels - 33% had concentrations of more than 14 µmol/l and 24% more than 15 µmol/l, while none of the healthy age- and sex-matched white control group had levels in excess of 14 µmol/l. The mean homocysteine level in the control group was 8.49 µmol/l (range: 4.35-13.92 µmol/l). Although genetic and dietary factors may be implicated, the elevated homocysteine levels nevertheless reflect increased risk of heart disease in this group.

6.4   **Conclusion**

It is likely that fortification of food with folic acid would lower plasma homocysteine levels in at least some sections of the general population of the United Kingdom. Observational studies suggest that this might in turn reduce the incidence of cardiovascular disease. However, although observational studies indicate a positive relationship between blood homocysteine levels and risk of cardiovascular disease, the interpretation of such studies can be problematical, and estimates of the magnitude of the relationship vary widely. In the absence of more definitive evidence linking folate intake directly with cardiovascular disease, it would not be justifiable at present to advocate dietary fortification with folic acid solely with the aim of reducing the incidence of cardiovascular disease. Clearly, however, cardiovascular diseases are such common causes of death and disability that if the projections from observational studies are accurate, fortification of food with folic acid would be of widespread benefit in the population.

7. Folate/folic acid: neurolo and neuropsychiatric asp

7.1 Background

The concentration of folate in the form of methylfolate in the cerebrospinal fluid is approximately three times higher than that in the serum. Through the homocysteine/methionine pathway and ultimately through S-adenosylmethionine, methylfolate provides the methyl group in innumerable methylation reactions in the nervous system, involving, for example, nucleoproteins, proteins, phospholipids, monoamines and neurotransmitters. Methylfolate may also influence monoamine metabolism and mood through the biopterin pathway[107].

7.2 Neurological and neuropsychiatric disorders

7.2.1 Impairments of both folate status and vitamin B_{12} status can lead to neurological and neuropsychiatric disorders. There is a poor correlation between the haematological and the neurological/neuropsychiatric manifestations of either folate or vitamin B_{12} deficiency. The biochemical mechanisms underlying the haematological and nervous system complications of folate and vitamin B_{12} may be different[108].

7.2.2 The neurological and neuropsychiatric manifestations of folate and vitamin B_{12} deficiencies, like the haematological manifestations, overlap considerably, and include cognitive impairment, mood disorders, subacute combined degeneration (SCD) and peripheral neuropathy. A classical neurological complication of vitamin B_{12} deficiency is SCD, which is invariably accompanied by peripheral neuropathy. However, it is less common in modern medical practice, probably owing to the earlier detection and treatment of deficiency states. SCD is very rare with folate deficiency[14,109]. Today, the commonest association with vitamin B_{12} deficiency is peripheral neuropathy, and with folate deficiency it is mood disorder. Both deficiencies lead to a similar amount of cognitive impairment[110]. About a third of patients with severe deficiencies of either vitamin, for example leading to megaloblastic anaemia, may have no detectable neuropsychiatric disorder. Likewise, other patients may present with neurological and neuropsychiatric disorders with little or no evidence of megaloblastic anaemia[111].

7.2.3 The neuropathology of the myeloneuropathy of vitamin B_{12} or rarely folate deficiency includes axonal degeneration and demyelination, especially in the posterior and lateral columns of the spinal cord[109,111]. Demyelination has also been observed in the cerebral lesions, including in children with inborn errors of vitamin B_{12} and folate metabolism[107].

.4   The neurological and neuropsychiatric manifestations of folate and
vitamin B_{12} deficiency may respond to appropriate vitamin therapy[109], but the
degree of response will vary with the severity and especially the duration of the
disorder and also the age of the patient. The older the patient, the less the potential
for recovery. Early diagnosis and treatment are essential at all ages, especially
in older people. Improvement can continue for a year or more[107,111].

7.3   Neuropsychiatric disorders and folate deficiency

Low or borderline red cell folate has been found in up to one-third of psychiatric
admissions and in an even higher proportion of psycho-geriatric patients[112],
sometimes but not always as the result of a poor diet due to mental illness.
Whether primary or secondary, clinical trials[107,113] have shown that such patients
respond less well to psychotropic medication and, conversely, respond to a
significantly greater degree after improvement of folate status.

7.4   Epilepsy

Several of the older anti-epileptic drugs (phenobarbitone, phenytoin, primidone)
can lead to folate deficiency in patients with epilepsy[108]. The degree of deficiency
is related to the dosage and, to some extent, the duration of exposure to the
drugs. Folate deficiency in epileptic subjects is associated with neuropsychiatric
disorders, but the correction of the deficiency has been reported to be associated
in some uncontrolled trials with an increase in seizures[108]. Patients receiving
phenytoin for epilepsy may have convulsions on large doses of folic acid, which
both decrease the drug's concentration in the cerebrospinal fluid and
experimentally increase excitatory effects[114]. There is a significant risk of fetal
abnormalities, including neural tube defects, associated with all the standard
epileptic drugs, including carbamazepine and sodium valproate, which have little
or no known effect on folate metabolism but have an effect on the glycine
clearance system for which folate is a cofactor[115]. Sodium valproate has been
most widely incriminated in causing neural tube defect.

7.5   Dementia

Low serum vitamin B_{12} without anaemia has been detected in up to 5% of
psychiatric admissions and up to 10% or more of psycho-geriatric or elderly
populations. Recent studies[107,116] involving additional techniques (CSF folate,
plasma homocysteine, plasma methyl malonic acid) have confirmed these
deficiency states in psychiatric and elderly populations, and suggest that they
may contribute to cognitive decline (dementia) in older people.

8. Other possible effects increasing folic acid in.

8.1 Anaemia

8.1.1 Folate is essential for DNA synthesis. Deficiency of this vitamin particularly affects rapidly dividing tissues such as bone marrow and mucous membranes, leading to symptoms of anaemia and sore tongue. The diagnosis is based on macrocytic red blood cells and hypersegmented neutrophils in the peripheral blood, on typical morphological changes of megaloblastosis in bone marrow, on low concentrations of folate in serum and red blood cells, and on the exclusion of vitamin B_{12} deficiency. Folate deficiency is usually due to poor diet, and it is also more likely during periods of increased need, such as pregnancy. It occurs with malabsorption, e.g. gluten-induced enteropathy. Treatment with synthetic folic acid is rapidly effective in reversing this picture.

8.1.2 Vitamin B_{12} (cobalamin) deficiency causes morphological changes in the bone marrow and red blood cells identical to those seen with folate deficiency, while the distinguishing feature is a low serum vitamin B_{12} level. In addition, a proportion of cases manifests neurological disorders, which sometimes include subacute combined degeneration of the spinal cord (SCD). The neuropathy may be so severe as to leave the individual chairbound and can be irreversible. Pernicious anaemia (PA) is the major cause of vitamin B_{12} deficiency in the UK and probably accounts for 80% of cases of megaloblastic anaemia. PA is an autoimmune disease, which destroys the gastric parietal cells that secrete intrinsic factor, which is necessary for the absorption of vitamin B_{12} in the terminal ileum. Patients who may have other causes of severe vitamin B_{12} deficiency, e.g. total gastrectomy, ileal resection, the rare intestinal blind loop syndrome or inborn errors of vitamin B_{12} absorption or transport, should be given prophylactic vitamin B_{12} therapy. Vitamin B_{12} can be absorbed by mechanisms independent of intrinsic factor, but high doses are required. Veganism rarely leads to vitamin B_{12} deficiency of sufficient severity to cause vitamin B_{12} neuropathy.

8.1.3 The metabolism of vitamin B_{12} and that of folate are closely related (para 2.4.3). The mechanism by which vitamin B_{12} deficiency causes megaloblastic anaemia is through its effect on folate metabolism with consequent inhibition of DNA synthesis. The severity of anaemia in severe vitamin B_{12} deficiency is related to the patient's folate status, those with higher serum and red cell folate levels being less likely to have anaemia. All patients with vitamin B_{12} neuropathy are severely vitamin B_{12}-deficient as assessed by serum vitamin B_{12} levels, but anaemia may be absent. If patients with vitamin B_{12} deficiency receive folic acid, the anaemia may be ameliorated, but there is a risk that the diagnosis of vitamin B_{12} deficiency may, as a result, be delayed, so increasing the possibility of the development of neuropathy.

Folate and vitamin B$_{12}$ inter-relations

.1   Several studies from the 1940s and 1950s showed this initial favourable response with later relapse and the development of neuropathy in a proportion of those being treated with folic acid, usually in daily doses of 5 mg or more. Neuropathy developed in a variable proportion of patients over months or years. The most serious complication, which was sometimes described as leading to explosive deterioration, was SCD. It has been suggested that administration of these high doses of folic acid might have precipitated neurological degeneration. Schwartz et al[117] treated 85 patients with PA with 5 mg of folic acid daily. After 3½ years: 23 (27%) had a haematological relapse, 23 (27%) neurological relapse, and a further 9 (11%) mixed neurological and haematological relapse. Wagley[118] treated 10 cases of PA with 15-30 mg folic acid daily for up to 1 year, during which time eight developed a neuropathy. Will et al[119] treated 36 PA patients for 1-10 years with folic acid at doses >1.0 mg daily: 21 (59%) showed a neurological relapse, and a further 9 (25%) combined haematological and neurological relapse. Israels & Wilkinson[120] found that 13 (65%) of 20 PA patients developed neuropathy while receiving folic acid and, in a further 3 (15%), neuropathy became worse.

8.2.2   The British National Formulary acknowledges a possible risk of high doses of folic acid. Clinicians in practice 40 years ago were convinced that patients with vitamin B$_{12}$ deficiency were at increased risk of SCD, which could progress rapidly if they were treated with a high dose of folic acid, because:

i.   the incidence of vitamin B$_{12}$ neuropathy was high (up to 80%) within one year of commencing folic acid in untreated vitamin B$_{12}$ deficiency;

ii.   there appeared to be a particularly high possibility of severe neurological symptoms developing at about three months after starting folic acid in these patients;

iii.   there was some evidence of a higher incidence of neuropathy as the dose of folic acid increased from 1.0 mg to 15 mg or more daily.

8.2.3   It is now not possible to prove whether or not there is an increased rate of SCD, or whether the neuropathy is made more severe as a result of giving folic acid to vitamin B$_{12}$-deficient individuals. Such a study would be unethical. Although folic acid is not toxic to normal individuals even in large doses, it might appear to be neurotoxic in the special circumstance of vitamin B$_{12}$ deficiency. Without a comparable control group, the issue must remain uncertain. It is generally agreed that there are no data that demonstrate that folic acid is harmful to the nervous system in people with vitamin B$_{12}$ deficiency at doses of 1 mg/day or less in the short term.

8.2.4   There is no suggestion that doses even higher than this might have adverse effects in the absence of vitamin B$_{12}$ deficiency. Nevertheless, folic acid can correct the anaemia of vitamin B$_{12}$ deficiency in some patients even at doses less than 1 mg/day, although this effect diminishes with decreasing dose (para 2.4.4). This could alter the presentation of vitamin B_{12} deficiency in the population (with a larger proportion of patients presenting with altered sensation and a smaller proportion presenting symptoms of anaemia). It is not possible to predict the effect on the incidence of irreversible vitamin B_{12} neuropathy, although arguments can be put forward to suggest it might increase owing to a delay in the diagnosis, which can depend on detecting the anaemia. Any general policy to increase dietary folic acid consumption should require vigilance with regard to the incidence, prevalence and presentation of vitamin B_{12} neuropathy in the community to determine whether these change.

8.2.5   A survey of 16 million people registered with General Practitioners in the UK showed a prevalence of PA of 127 per 100,000 population[121]. It is a disease of later life as only 11% of PA cases present before the age of 40. In Glasgow, the prevalence of PA was shown to be 1% in people over the age of 60 increasing to 2-5% in over 65 year olds. In north west England, 3.7% of people aged over 75 were diagnosed with PA[122,123]. There may be a substantial number of older people in whom pernicious anaemia remains undiagnosed. A small study in the USA[124] in 729 people aged 60 years and over found that 14 (1.9%, 95% CI 1.41%-2.43%) without diagnosed PA had antibodies to intrinsic factor. However, only 9 of these 14 (1.2%) had subnormal serum vitamin B_{12} levels. If the prevalences are similar in the UK, around 150,000 people aged over 60 years with unrecognised vitamin B_{12} deficiency could be at risk if exposed to high intakes of folic acid. As noted earlier, older people are already exposed to unregulated intakes of folic acid through voluntary fortification of breakfast cereals. Moreover, manufacturers usually add more folic acid than is necessary to achieve the minimum level specified in order to compensate for losses during manufacture and storage of fortified foods. If fortification continues to be unregulated, it is possible that older people with undiagnosed PA would be at a greater hazard from vitamin B_{12} deficiency. Vitamin B_{12} neuropathy is more frequent in males with an incidence ratio of 10M:7F, although pernicious anaemia is more common in females (1.6F:1M)[123]. The vitamin B_{12} status of a group of people representative of the British population aged 65 years or older is shown in Table 8.1.

Table 8.1 Proportion of a large group of older people representative of the British population with poor cobalamin status[11] [assessed as proportion with mean corpuscular volume (MCV)>101fl and proportion with serum vitamin B_{12} <118 pmol/l (160 ng/l)]

Age (yrs) and gender	Not living in institution		Living in institution	
	MCV >101fl	Serum vitamin B_{12} <118 pmol/l (160 ng/l)	MCV >101fl	Serum vitamin B_{12} <118 pmol/l (160 ng/l)
	n = 489 %	n = 480 %	n = 144 %	n = 142 %
Men				
65-74	2	6	}	}
75-84	3	11	}2	}9
85+	1	10	8	4
All 65+	2	8	4	7
	n = 461	n = 456	n = 134	n = 122
Women				
65-74	3	2	}	}
75-84	1	9	}1	}8
85+	2	10	4	11
All 65+	3	5	3	10

n = number in the group

8.2.6   In addition to its role in preventing anaemia and neurological damage, vitamin B_{12} has been shown to influence homocysteine levels. The homocysteine-lowering potential of a folic acid supplement was compared with that of supplements containing different doses of vitamin B_{12} in addition to folic acid[125]. In this study, 150 women of childbearing age were given a placebo initially for 4 weeks followed by a 4-week treatment period of either 400 µg of folic acid or 400 µg of folic acid + 6 µg of vitamin B_{12} or 400 µg of folic acid + 400 µg of vitamin B_{12}. Significant reductions in plasma homocysteine levels were observed in all groups, but the reduction with supplements containing vitamin B_{12} was larger than that with folic acid alone (-11%). Folic acid in combination with 6 µg of vitamin B_{12} reduced homocysteine levels by 15% while a reduction of 18% was observed in the group that received 400 µg of vitamin B_{12}.

8.2.7   As there is no known toxicity of vitamin B_{12}, it may be feasible to add high levels during fortification, if it is shown to be practical. There have been several calls for such a policy to be introduced, particularly in the USA, where a lower level of fortification with folic acid was adopted to prevent NTDs taking into consideration the problems of possible vitamin B_{12} deficiency[126,127]. It would be necessary to fortify foods with high levels of vitamin B_{12} (in order to achieve intakes of around 100-1000 μg/day) to allow for the low absorption in older people with pernicious anaemia, which is the primary cause of vitamin B_{12} deficiency in this group. The implications of such high intakes of vitamin B_{12} by the general population are not known. Moreover, there is a possibility of problems with the diagnosis of vitamin B_{12} deficiency due to the appearance of various vitamin B_{12} analogues in blood when an abnormally large amount of vitamin B_{12} is present in the food supply.

8.3   Cancer

It has been suggested that low intakes of folate might increase the risk of cancer in man. A long-term study in about 90,000 nurses reported that the relative risk for colon cancer was markedly lower (0.25, 95% CI 0.13-0.51) after 15 years in those who reported using multivitamin supplements containing folic acid. The investigators concluded that the effect might be related to the folic acid contained in multivitamins. However, the supplement users were self-selected, which may introduce bias, and folate/folic acid intakes in the study were measured using semi-quantitative food frequency questionnaires and therefore any associations should be interpreted with caution[128]. In 1998, COMA[129] concluded that there was insufficient evidence for any specific links between folate intake and the development of cancer.

9. Issues relating to fortification with folic acid

9.1 General concepts of risk

9.1.1 *Risk assessment*

"Risk", or the chance of something (usually adverse) happening, can be considered in terms of a consequence, and of its likelihood. There may be diverse consequences (or hazards), each with different likelihoods (or risks). Where the consequence is known, the statistical probability of its occurring can be calculated from population data - for example, the risk of lung cancer in miners working in regions of high natural radioactivity. This "assessment of risk", which is conducted by experts, takes account of the available scientific data. The risk is usually presented as falling within a range of probability, which will narrow as more data are collected.

9.1.2 *Perception of risk*

These are familiar concepts for scientists but not for the majority of the general public. For this and other reasons, the estimate of risk derived by scientific calculations may not be accepted unquestioningly[130]. Other powerful influences, such as peer group pressure or personal experience, shape the perception of the individual. For example, most people are horrified by a train crash however minor, yet road traffic casualties are accepted as a consequence of modern life. The dread which a defined risk poses is perceived differently depending on, for instance, how much control individuals may have over the risk, and the degree of uncertainty over its nature or size, or the nature of the hazard. The term "risk management" has been used to describe the ways in which risk is dealt with taking account of these different perspectives. Some of the factors that commonly influence people's perception of risk are listed in the Department of Health publication "Communicating about Risks to Public Health 1997"[131].

9.1.3 *The balance of risk*

There are few situations where all the risks are adverse. For example, areas of high flood risk may have particularly fertile soil. Where some consequences are good and some bad, the term balance of risk is used to describe the overall experience. Sometimes, both the adverse and beneficial consequences are borne by the same group. In other cases, one group may experience the benefit while another carries the risk. Each situation therefore needs to be assessed on its merits.

9.2 Risks associated with food

9.2.1 The usual understanding of food risks concerns hazards such as chemical, biological or physical agents in food. Examples are dioxins, bacterial contamination such as *Salmonella* or radionuclides. In these cases, there is no direct benefit from consuming these agents, although the food itself may be an important dietary component. The ideal would be complete absence of the agents, although this may not be feasible for technical, economic, or other reasons. In other cases, the agent may have benefits that are seen as desirable for a variety of reasons but not essential, such as an additive to colour food, a pesticide applied during growth to enhance the crop, or a preservative to improve the shelf-life of a food. Toxicological assessment attempts to identify, for such substances, the levels of exposure that minimise the risk of adverse effects.

9.2.2 *Risk and nutrients*

Nutrients are chemical agents in food which have a structural or metabolic function in the body. It is possible not to get enough, or to get too much. The traditional risk of getting too little is the basis of the derivation of population Dietary Reference Values. Manipulating the diet through fortification and dietary supplements increases the possibility of exposure unwittingly to undesirably high levels of some micronutrients. Safety margins (the gap between the necessary level of intake and levels carrying a risk of adverse effects) for the fat-soluble vitamins A and D were identified over 30 years ago. Other micronutrients may also have adverse effects at high intakes. The USA has recently defined a Tolerable Upper Intake Level as the highest daily nutrient intake that is likely to pose no risks of adverse health effects to almost all individuals in the general population[25]. Additionally, inappropriate intakes of energy and of individual macronutrients, such as fat, can increase the risk of chronic diseases. It is more difficult to define precisely the balance of macronutrients that is or is not associated with a defined health outcome, although the public health significance of such factors may be substantial.

9.3 Folic acid and risk

9.3.1 The proven benefits of folic acid supplementation are in the small group of women who might otherwise have offspring with neural tube defects. Adverse effects of folic acid have been proposed to be associated with deficiency of vitamin B_{12}, itself not usually due to dietary causes and generally affecting older population groups. On the other hand, there may be a benefit on vascular or mental health in the same group from additional folate which is largely independent of the status of other nutrients. In addition, average folate status of people aged 65 years or over is low as assessed against conventional criteria (para 3.7.2). An increase in dietary folate intake would be a benefit in this respect, at least in traditional nutritional terms. The different hazards, and the different groups that might experience them, together with uncertainty over the benefits and over their size, make an overall assessment difficult. Other factors also give cause for prudence in assessing safety. For instance, adverse effects are not usually reported in systematic reviews[132], and others may emerge only decades later[133].

9.3.2 *Risk assessment applied to folate/folic acid*

The adverse consequences of inadequate folate on haemopoiesis and on mucous membranes have been known for over 50 years. This Report addresses the more recently identified risk of neural tube defect from an inadequate intake, and also evaluates available data on the risk of adverse effects from excessive intake, especially when given as folic acid supplements, which is a synthetic and more bioavailable form of the vitamin. It is reassuring to note that, in the USA, increasing intakes of folic acid from fortified foods and increased use of dietary supplements have not been accompanied by a reported increase in adverse effects. On the other hand, the monitoring of adverse effects which might be attributed to increasing intakes of folic acid may not be comprehensive. Given the paucity of data, judgement must inevitably contribute in large measure to any risk assessment in relation to increasing folic acid intakes.

9.4   **Involving interest groups**

9.4.1   Society as a whole has to retain confidence in the food it eats, and modification of a staple food, even for intended health benefit, should be undertaken only after appropriate involvement of the public. The following aspects are important.

a.   Public education   There is much to be gained from involving the public in decisions taken on public health grounds. Although public opinion, at least as expressed and manipulated by the media, is often regarded as capricious, most people are reasonable. Public education allows informed participation in the debate. Understanding of the benefits of increased folate/folic acid intakes for women of childbearing age was enhanced by the Health Education Authority Folic Acid Campaign in 1995-7 (Annex 2). The possible risk from excess to older people has not yet been addressed by any health promotion campaigns. Education about possible risks to older people would help in developing publicly acceptable policy.

b.   Public confidence in continued monitoring   Understanding of the nature and extent of risks and benefits involved in any new policy can never be complete. Policies, such as fortifying a staple food, therefore require acceptance not only by policy makers but also by potential beneficiaries, and by potential risk bearers. Continued monitoring for both benefit and adverse effects is an important contribution. Confidence in the quality of technology that is being employed is also important.

c.   The public's right to know   Efforts must be made to provide the public with information in an easily accessible and understandable form. The labelling of loaves and other fortified products should ensure that the relevant nutrition information is provided in an easily understandable form. The public should be informed of the results of health monitoring or other relevant scientific data. New data may change the balance of risks, and this should also be communicated.

9.4.2   Fortification of foods with folic acid carries some benefits that are certain, others that are less certain, and the possibility of adverse effects. These beneficial and adverse effects fall on different groups in the population. Consequently, determining the overall balance of advantage and disadvantage from a population-wide exposure is not straightforward. The public has a right to know the composition of food, and that it is safe, and to contribute to debates about public health policy relating to it. Ultimately, decisions on public health policy are the responsibility of Ministers, who need to have as full information as possible about the consequences of the various options available to them.

9.5   Possible strategies for fortification of foods

9.5.1   An increase in folic acid intakes would help prevent NTDs and lower homocysteine levels in blood, which might contribute to reducing the risk of cardiovascular disease. Theoretically, an increase in folic acid intakes could be achieved through diet (but in practice it is likely to be difficult unless large amounts of single sources of folate - for example, Brussels sprouts or broccoli - are consumed) or by supplementation and/or fortification of staple foods such as flour. With any of the methods, it is essential to deliver the appropriate dose to the appropriate target group and ensure maximum benefit to public health at a minimum risk of adverse effects from high intakes in vulnerable groups. The USA has approved a policy of food fortification in which folic acid is added at a level of 140 μg/100 g of grain, estimated to achieve an additional mean intake of 100 μg of folic acid per day with an expected maximum of 1000 μg. The efficacy of the fortification level in the USA is still being debated.

9.5.2   Recognising that women with red-cell folate concentrations above 400 μg/l are at very low risk of NTD births, Daly et al[50] studied the effect of supplements of 100 μg, 200 μg and 400 μg in a placebo-controlled trial involving 172 women with red-cell folate levels initially between 150 μg/l and 400 μg/l. The median changes in red-cell folate in all women who completed the trial were –12, 67, 130 and 200 μg/l in the placebo, 100, 200 and 400 mg in the supplementation groups, respectively. The reductions in risk for NTD conceptions that would be associated with these changes were estimated, on the basis of a case-control study[134], to be 22%, 41% and 47%, respectively. The supplement study was short-term and the majority of women receiving supplements at any level were in positive folate balance, suggesting that benefits of continued increased folate intakes might increase over time.

9.5.3   The inverse relationship between red-cell folate and birth prevalence of NTD is continuous and follows a power-law function over the range for which data are available[91]. In broad terms, a 40% increase in red-cell folate is associated with around a 30% decrease in birth prevalence of NTD. There is no evidence of a ceiling above which increases in red-cell folate cease to confer further benefit, but in terms of the numbers rather than the percentages of NTDs prevented by each increment, the relationship is one of diminishing returns. Public health policy is a matter of achieving a compromise between increasing the folate intake of women becoming pregnant to as high a level as possible without exposing other sections of the population to hazard. As Daly et al[135] point out, in addition to concerns over the effects of folic acid on people with undiagnosed pernicious anaemia, there are no data on the safety of prolonged exposure of children to doses above 1 mg a day.

9.5.4   For obvious reasons, the aim of public health policy is to reduce the number of NTD conceptions rather than to provide only for termination of affected pregnancies. Unfortunately, we have no good data on the numbers of affected conceptions since, as already discussed, many abort spontaneously and there is known to be significant under-reporting of the numbers of therapeutic terminations of pregnancies that are affected by NTD, but estimates for the UK range from 600-1200 per year[61,62]. The only reasonably reliable data that we have are the numbers of affected live and still births and, even with these, there probably is a degree of under-reporting. Ninety three NTD-affected births were reported in 1998 in England and Wales, and in 1997, 65 in Scotland and 14 in Northern Ireland (Annex 5). Clearly, however, policy makers and the public need to have some idea of the expected magnitude of benefits to be derived from a global modification of the national food supply.

9.5.5   In Table 9.1, we present the best estimates we have been able to derive on the effect of increasing folic acid intake through fortification of flour at different levels (para 9.5.9, Tables A7.1, A7.2) on the numbers of births affected by NTDs using the latest available data from England and Wales. The figures presented must not be regarded as anything more than broad indicators of the magnitude of likely effects. While the relationship between red-cell folate and risk of NTD is reasonably well established, that between folate intake and red cell level is hard to characterise because of the difficulties in measuring dietary intake. For the effect on median red-cell folate of increasing folate intake we have only the three data points provided by the 100-, 200- and 400 µg supplements used by Daly et al[50]. For the estimates of NTDs in Table 9.1 we have used linear interpolation between these three points as there are no a priori grounds for adopting more sophisticated mathematical models. The underlying relationship is presumably continuous; however, linear interpolation assumes that, over the range of 100 to 200 µg additional dietary folate, red-cell folate rises by around 1 µg/l per dietary 1 µg, but over the range 200 to 400 µg by only 0.3 µg/l per dietary 1 µg. The critical point of inflection occurs at the modelled fortification level of 240 µg/100 g of flour as this corresponds to a mean additional daily intake of 201 µg of folic acid. The major part of potential benefit in reducing NTD incidence seems attainable at or above this level of fortification, but the predicted effects on NTD incidence of varying levels around this point are too uncertain to provide a basis for policy. The limiting consideration becomes the possible hazard of high intakes by some sections of the community, as discussed later.

Table 9.1   Estimates of number of NTD births prevented in England and Wales at different fortification levels based on estimates from Daly et al[50] and data on folic acid intakes in 16-45 year old women from the Dietary and Nutritional Survey of British Adults[32] (Annex 6).

Fortification level μg/100 g of flour	Average additional FA intake μg/day	Average total intake folate+FA μg/day	% Reduction in risk	No. of NTD births prevented based on current level of 93/yr (1998)*
-	100[+]	-	22[+]	-
140	117	321	25	23
200	167	371	35	32
240	201	405	41	38
280	234	438	42	39
420	351	555	46	42
-	400[+]	-	47[+]	-

[+] The number of NTDs that would be prevented under different fortification scenarios has been estimated using the data on the percentage reduction of risk reported by Daly et al[50] on delivery of 100, 200 and 400 μg/day of folic acid in fortified foods (paras 9.5.2 to 9.5.5). The calculations should be interpreted with caution because:

the baseline folate/folic acid intakes and folate status of the original sample are not known and could be different in the current UK population;

the reduction in risk might not be the same, as it might depend on baseline folate status and, if the status has since improved, there could be a modest overestimation of reduction in risk;

the estimated proportionate reduction in NTD births might differ owing to other factors.

* Source: National Congenital Anomaly System, Office for National Statistics[60]

9.5.6   The effect of fortification on plasma homocysteine levels has been addressed in two trials using fortified breakfast cereals. Fortified breakfast cereal containing folic acid was given to men and women to deliver daily doses of 127 μg or 499 μg or 665 μg in a double blind placebo-controlled crossover trial[48]. Plasma folate and homocysteine levels were measured initially and after 5 weeks of supplementation. An additional intake of 127 μg/day reduced plasma homocysteine levels by 3.7% and higher intakes of 499 μg/day and 665 μg/day reduced homocysteine levels by 11% and 14%, respectively. An intervention trial by Schorah et al[49] in men and women used breakfast cereals fortified with folic acid to provide a level of 200 μg/day with or without other multivitamins for 24 weeks. There was a significant reduction (10%) in homocysteine levels in groups that received fortified cereals compared with the placebo group. The effect of folic acid fortification on reducing plasma homocysteine levels was significantly greater (p=0.001) in those subjects who began the study with lowest serum folate levels. Folic acid supplementation did not affect homocysteine in those whose initial homocysteine levels were in the lowest tertile of the distribution, but had a significant impact in those in the mid and highest tertiles (p=0.006 and 0.005, respectively). This study is in agreement with that of Daly et al[50] and both suggest that 200 μg/day of extra folic acid can make an important contribution to reducing the metabolic disturbances associated with low folate status.

9.5.7   There are some early reports from the US on the effect of mandatory fortification on folate status in a sample of middle-aged and older people from the Framingham Offspring Study[93], in which the subjects undergo examinations approximately every 3 to 4 years. Baseline measurements in study (n=350) and control (n=756) groups were obtained before the implementation of fortification and follow-up measurements were made in the study group a few months after the introduction of fortification. In the case of the control group, follow-up measurements were obtained before the implementation of fortification. Folate status was measured by plasma folate and homocysteine levels; a low folate status was defined as a level less than 7 nmol/l and a high homocysteine level being greater than 13 μmol/l. The fortification of grain products with folic acid was associated with significant improvement in folate status and a significant decrease in homocysteine levels in those who did not use any vitamin B supplements. The proportion of subjects in the study group with low folate status decreased significantly (p<0.001) from 22% (95% CI 17.3-26.7%) to 1.7% (95% CI 0-5.4%). The prevalence of high homocysteine levels also decreased by 48% (p<0.001) from baseline to the follow-up examination. It is notable that the level of fortification at 140 μg/100 g in the US, predicted to provide an additional intake of 70-120 μg/day of folic acid to middle-aged and older adults resulted in a substantial decrease in homocysteine levels. However, other experimental studies[48] have concluded that an additional intake of 100 μg/day of folic acid was not sufficient to lower homocysteine levels. It is possible that grain products are being fortified at higher than the required level of folic acid, which could have resulted in such a substantial decrease in homocysteine levels in the population. There is little information on the amount of overage that is added during fortification to overcome any loss of folic acid during processing and storage of food products.

9.5.8   The prevailing intakes of folate/folic acid in the UK diet (an average of 250 μg/day) are below those recommended to minimise risk of NTD in women of childbearing age, namely 600 μg daily. In addition, a number of people in other sections of the population, in particular older people, do not consume folate/folic acid at a level estimated to meet their requirements, based on existing DRV, and biochemical markers of folate status are also low in this group. The information on supplement use in women of childbearing age is from dietary information collected in 1986/87 and is likely to underestimate their current usage, while that in older age groups is more recent, based on data collected in 1994/95. Higher folate intakes can be achieved either by individual decisions to take dietary supplements of folic acid or eat foods rich in natural folates or fortified with folic acid, or by more generally fortifying the food supply to increase intakes in the population as a whole. An increase of 400 μg of folic acid in addition to the current folate intake would reduce the risk of NTDs substantially (by an estimated 47-53%). This intake of more than 600 μg/day of total folate could not reasonably be achieved without fortification or by more widespread use of supplements. The most appropriate staple food for fortification would be flour and breakfast cereals because of their near universal consumption and relatively narrow variability of consumption in the population. An intake of 600 μg/day of total folate by all women of childbearing age cannot be achieved through folic acid fortification of flour without exposing a substantial number of older people, aged 50 and over, to intakes above 1 mg/day (Table A7.2).

9.5.9   In considering possible strategies for fortification in the UK, several scenarios were investigated to assess the likely impact on folate intakes in different sexes and age groups. The food consumption data from the latest NDNS surveys in each age group have been used for the analyses and the most recent data on folate from the food composition tables have been applied. The fieldwork for the NDNS survey of British adults aged 16-64 years was conducted in 1986/87, and the use of dietary supplements is likely to have changed in this group. The estimated folate intakes used in the modelling exercise do not take into account within-individual (day-to-day) variation in intakes. Four different levels of fortification, at 140, 200, 240 and 280 μg/100 g of all flour and of flour with the exclusion of wholemeal, were calculated. The possible exemption of wholemeal flour might have different implications for different groups in the population, especially if certain groups consume more of their flour in the wholemeal form. The exemption of wholemeal flour was found to have little influence on folate intakes of manual classes but a relatively greater impact on non-manual classes in the population. Since only 1% of the total flour used in the UK is imported, it was not separately considered, and is likely to exert little influence on the hypothetical results generated from the modelling exercise set out in Tables A7.1 and A7.2. The levels of fortification were chosen initially as multiples of amounts necessary for restoring the amount of total folate in white flour to its original level (as in wholemeal flour). In addition, the current levels of fortification (140 μg/100 g) in other countries, such as the USA and Australia, were also taken into consideration. Wholemeal flour contains 60-70 μg/100 g of folate. The estimated total folate intakes in the model include the amount of folic acid currently provided by voluntary fortification of foods such as breakfast cereals and dietary supplements. The levels of fortification were calculated as folate present in the foods as consumed.

9.5.10   After careful consideration of predicted benefits and possible hazards, we have appraised some options for action. The appraisal of options balances the predicted benefits to younger women, protecting them from NTD conceptions, against possible adverse effects such as neuropathy, especially in older people who might have vitamin B_{12} deficiency. Our calculations of the benefits and possible hazards, and the balance between them, have been based on modelling the expected exposure of different age and sex groups to folate, at different levels of fortification of flour and at current levels of voluntary fortification of breakfast cereals. We have assumed target levels of fortification such that the level is precisely maintained in the food supply over a reasonable period of time. Current practice in fortifying foods is to ensure that the amount of fortificant in the product as purchased is not less than the amount claimed on the label. To ensure that levels do not fall below such a minimum, manufacturers usually add more nutrients than necessary (overage) to take account of losses during processing and storage. However, if such an overage were used in fortifying foods with folic acid, this would exceed the target level, and people would be exposed to higher than expected levels. Unfortunately, the degree of overage is highly variable, and no research has been done on the ability of industry to deliver a target (as opposed to a minimum) level. Such uncertainty raises difficulties for embodying a target level in a safe and effective policy. Whichever option is chosen, there should be continued monitoring of rates of NTD occurrence, and clinical vigilance, especially in older people, with the aim of early detection of vitamin B_{12} deficiency. In addition, there should be regular monitoring of fortification levels in bread and other products containing flour.

9.6   Options for action

9.6.1   The options for action suggested below are based on data available at the present time and should not be regarded as permanent solutions. Any policy should be reviewed in the future in the light of changes in the prevailing situation.

Option 1   *Continue or intensify education programme without universal fortification*

The success of the Folic Acid Campaign in raising the awareness of women planning to become pregnant with regard to the importance of increasing folic acid intakes argues for the continuation, and possibly intensification, of the programme. Monitoring of rates of NTD and changes in the uptake of termination of pregnancies should provide the basis for evaluating the effectiveness of the education programme. The probability of vitamin B_{12} deficiency being undetected in some groups, particularly older people, as a consequence of increased intake of folic acid *via* general fortification will be avoided, but the present unregulated fortification practices allow the possibility of inadvertent excess or deficiency to continue. This option, taken alone, is unlikely to increase folic acid intake amongst the proportion of women whose pregnancies are unplanned, or to benefit the group of older people whose folate/folic acid intakes remain low. However, this option is not exclusive of other options, and there would be advantage in continuing existing education whatever other policies might also be adopted.

Option 2   *Fortification at 140 µg/100 g of flour*

Fortification at a level of 140 µg/100 g of flour is estimated to increase folic acid intake by an average of 117 µg/day in women of childbearing age, but 99% would have total intakes <600 µg/day. This option is not likely to have the maximum achievable effect on the prevention of NTDs. However, there are theoretical reasons[50] why even this relatively small increase in folic acid consumption might decrease risk of NTD more than might be expected, even though only a quarter of the target extra intake of 400 µg of folic acid is met. Based on data relating folic acid intake to folate status and folate status to risk, it is estimated (Table 9.1) that such an intake might achieve about one-third of the maximum possible benefit - around 25% reduction in risk compared with 65-75% maximum theoretically achievable. This would translate into an estimated reduction of about 22 NTD-affected births per year. This option would need to be considered with continuing public education of the need for women who might become pregnant to take folic acid supplements, and to choose foods rich in folate/folic acid. However, fortification at this level is likely to avoid many of the potential problems of excess relating to vitamin B_{12} deficiency in older people. It is estimated that 0.1% of people aged 50 and above might be exposed to intakes of over 1000 µg/day (Table A7.2).

Option 3   *Fortification at 200 µg/100 g of flour*

Fortification at a level of 200 µg/100 g of flour is estimated to increase folic acid intake by an average of 167 µg/day in women of childbearing age, but 97% would have total intakes <600 µg/day. This option is not likely to have the maximum possible effect on the prevention of NTDs. However, even this increase in folic acid consumption, which is half of the target additional intake of 400 µg/day, might decrease risk of NTD[50]. Based on data relating folic acid intake to folate status and folate status to risk, it is estimated (Table 9.1) that such an intake might achieve about 35% reduction in risk, compared with 65-75% maximum theoretically achievable. This would translate into an estimated reduction of about 32 fewer NTD-affected births per year. This option would need to be considered with continuing public education of the need for women who might become pregnant to take folic acid supplements, and to choose foods rich in folate/folic acid. However, fortification at this level is likely to avoid many of the potential problems of excess relating to vitamin B_{12} deficiency in older people. It is estimated that 0.2% of people aged 50 and above might be exposed to intakes of over 1000 µg/day (Table A7.2).

Option 4   *Fortification at 240 µg/100 g of flour*

This option is estimated to provide an average additional intake of folic acid of 201 µg/day to women aged 16-45 years, but 93% would have total folate intakes below 600 µg/day. This would be expected to reduce the risk of NTDs by about 41% (Table 9.1) compared with the maximum achievable of around 65-75%, resulting in 38 fewer births affected by NTD per year. These women need to continue taking folic acid supplements during pre- and peri-conception, and so the education programme should be continued. Our modelling indicates that about 0.6% of the 50+ age group might have intakes greater than 1000 µg/day, and the risk of undetected vitamin B_{12} deficiency in older people and potential adverse effects arising from it would require monitoring and clinical vigilance (Table A7.2). However, some people in this age group are also likely to benefit from an increase in folic acid as their current intakes are low.

Option 5   *Fortification at 280 µg/100 g of flour*

This option is estimated to provide an average additional intake of folic acid of 234 µg/day to women aged 16-45 years, but 87% of them would still have total folate intakes below 600 µg/day. This option is expected to reduce the risk of NTDs by about 42% - about two-thirds of the maximum achievable of 65-70%, and result in 39 fewer NTD-affected births per year (Table 9.1). Our modelling indicates that about 5% of men aged 50-64 years, but less than 1% of women aged over 50, and a total of 1.5% of all older people aged over 50 might have intakes greater than 1000 µg/day (Table A7.2). The risk of undetected vitamin B_{12} deficiency in older people and potential adverse effects arising from it would require monitoring and clinical vigilance. However, some people in this age group are also likely to benefit, as both their current intakes and folate status are poor. A reduction in circulating homocysteine levels, with the possibility of lowered cardiovascular risk and a beneficial effect in neurological function, are possible but as yet unproven. There should be heightened awareness amongst the medical profession to diagnose vitamin B_{12} deficiency in older people, and education programmes targeting women of childbearing age on the importance of folic acid, should continue.

Option 6 *Fortification at 420 µg/100 g of flour*

The higher level of fortification would provide an additional intake of folic acid of 351 µg/day and ensure that about 40% of women of childbearing age would achieve total folate intakes greater than 600 µg/day. The higher level of fortification would be expected to reduce the risk of NTD by about 46% compared with the maximum achievable of 65-75%, to result in 42 fewer NTD-affected births per year (Table 9.1). Around 9% of those in the older age group (50+) are calculated to have intakes greater than 1000 µg/day and a substantial minority might exceed 2000 µg/day (Table A7.2). In addition, approximately 60% of women of childbearing age would need to take supplements/fortified foods to achieve the recommended intake of 600 µg/day, and the public education campaign would need to be continued. The medical profession would need to exercise particular vigilance in respect of adverse effects in older people.

Option 7 *Combined fortification with folic acid and vitamin B_{12}*

In order to minimise the possibility of vitamin B_{12} deficiency, particularly in older people, the possibility and practicality of fortifying foods with vitamin B_{12} might be considered. There is no evidence of toxicity of vitamin B_{12} and, moreover, it has recently been shown that combined supplementation with both vitamins was efficacious in lowering circulating homocysteine levels (para 3.8.2). It would be necessary to fortify foods with very large amounts of vitamin B_{12} to allow for the low absorption in people with pernicious anaemia, which is the chief cause of severe deficiency. In addition, individual variation in the efficiency of absorption of vitamin B_{12} might influence the outcome. At present, there is inadequate information on the amount of vitamin B_{12} that would be required to ensure the absence of deficiency in the population, especially in those with pernicious anaemia. Although there is no formal evidence of toxicity from vitamin B_{12}, any exposure of the whole population to levels many times their usual intake or requirements should be considered with particular caution. In addition, technical aspects of fortification with high levels of vitamin B_{12} would have to be considered.

9.6.2 *Technical issues* We have modelled the likely exposures of various population groups on the basis of different levels of fortification of flour with folic acid, the level representing the amount in the food as consumed, and assuming no change in the intake of folic acid from other sources. A particular source of folic acid is breakfast cereals. However, as there are concerns not only about low, but also about excessive intake of folic acid, it is important to the eventual outcome that current levels of fortification of breakfast cereals do not change substantially. Any such change would make an important difference to the numbers of people exposed to different levels of folic acid, and so also to the balance of risk against benefit in the population as a whole. Consideration will need to be given to whether the levels of folic acid in breakfast cereals should be subject to some degree of control. Furthermore, these calculations are based on a precise content of folic acid in foods containing flour at the target level, and manufacturers will have to ensure that the target levels are maintained in flour products as consumed. However, for technical reasons, there is likely to be variation around this, and any decisions should take account of the ability of manufacturers not only to avoid unexpectedly low, but also undesirably high levels of folic acid in flour and its products.

9.6.3   On scientific, medical and public health grounds, the Committee concluded that universal folic acid fortification of flour at 240 µg/100 g of flour in foods as consumed would have a significant effect in preventing NTD-affected conceptions and births without resulting in unacceptably high intakes in any group of the population. However, any fortification policy should be reviewed in light of improving methodology in folate analysis and the emerging scientific knowledge on bioavailability of natural folates and folic acid from foods.

10. Conclusions

1. The risk of Neural Tube Defects (NTDs) can be reduced by increasing the intake of folic acid. There is an inverse dose response relationship between folate status and the risk of NTDs (Chapter 5). Current tentative estimates of recognised NTD pregnancies per year are in the range of 600-1200 in the UK. Consumption of 400 µg/day of folic acid in addition to a usual dietary intake of about 200 µg/day would be expected to reduce the risk of NTD by about a half.

2. These beneficial effects can be achieved through increasing intakes either of natural folate or of folic acid, but, as folic acid is more bio-available, it is likely to have a greater impact (Chapters 2 & 3).

3. All women who could become pregnant should continue to be advised to take 400 µg folic acid per day as a medicinal or food supplement prior to conception, and until the twelfth week of pregnancy. Women with a previous pregnancy affected by NTD, who wish to conceive, should be advised to take a daily supplement of 5 mg of folic acid (Chapter 1).

4. Higher total folate intakes can be achieved by individual decisions (to take dietary supplements of folic acid or eat foods rich in natural folates or fortified with folic acid) or by fortifying staple foods to increase intakes in the population (Chapter 9).

5. An intake of 600 µg/day of total folate (200 µg of natural folate + 400 µg of folic acid), by all women of childbearing age cannot be achieved through fortification of flour with folic acid without exposing a substantial number of older people to high intakes, which might be associated with adverse effects (Chapters 5, 8 & 9).

6. Increasing the intake of folate/folic acid might make vitamin B_{12} deficiency, particularly in the 50+ age group, less easy to detect by delaying the onset of anaemia. The possibility that prolonged intakes in excess of 1 mg/day might precipitate neuropathy in some people deficient in vitamin B_{12} cannot be discounted, but there is no evidence of adverse effects in women of childbearing age. There is a need for heightened clinical vigilance of vitamin B_{12} deficiency as a consequence of any increase in folic acid intakes, particularly in older people (Chapter 8).

7. Raised plasma homocysteine level is independently associated with the risk of occlusive vascular disease and possibly with the prevalence of certain neuropsychiatric disorders. There is an inverse graded relationship between

folate status and the circulating level of homocysteine. However, there is no evidence from randomised controlled trials that improving folate status, and thereby reducing homocysteine levels, will reduce the risk of cardiovascular disease or of neuropsychiatric problems in the population (Chapters 6 & 7).

8. The limited data available are insufficient to conclude that folate intake influences the development of colon or other cancers (Chapter 8).

9. Total folate intakes can be increased and homocysteine levels can be lowered through fortification of staple foods with folic acid (Chapters 8 & 9).

10. Estimates of the exposure of different groups in the population to additional folic acid were made by modelling dietary intake data from the latest NDNS surveys in each age group, at five levels of fortification of flour (including wholemeal) as consumed in finished products (Tables A7.1 & A7.2).

Fortification at 140 μg/100 g of flour

- The average intake of folic acid of women aged 16-45 years would increase by 117 μg/day, leading to an average total folate intake of 321 μg/day (Table 9.1).

- Approximately 0.7% of women in this age group would have total folate intakes in excess of 600 μg/day.

- It is estimated that 23 NTD-affected births per year would be prevented (Table 9.1).

- Approximately 0.1% of people aged over 50 years would be exposed to levels of folic acid intake greater than 1 mg/day (Table A7.2).

Fortification at 200 μg/100 g of flour

- The average intake of folic acid of women aged 16-45 years would increase by 167 μg/day, leading to a total folate intake of 371 μg/day (Table 9.1).

- Approximately 2.8% of women in this age group would have total folate intakes in excess of 600 μg/day.

- It is estimated that 32 NTD-affected births per year would be prevented (Table 9.1).

- Approximately 0.2% of people aged over 50 years would be exposed to levels of folic acid intake greater than 1 mg/day (Table A7.2).

Fortification at 240 µg/100 g of flour

- The average intake of folic acid of women aged 16-45 years would increase by 201 µg/day, leading to a total folate intake of 405 µg/day (Table 9.1).

- Approximately 7% of women in this age group would have total folate intakes in excess of 600 µg/day.

- It is estimated that 38 NTD-affected births per year would be prevented (Table 9.1).

- Approximately 0.6% of people aged over 50 years would be exposed to levels of folic acid intake greater than 1 mg/day (Table A7.2).

Fortification at 280 µg/100 g of flour

- The average intake of folic acid of women aged 16-45 years would increase by 234 µg/day, leading to a total folate intake of 438 µg/day (Table 9.1).

- Approximately 13% of women in this age group would have total folate intakes in excess of 600 µg/day.

- It is estimated that 39 NTD-affected births per year would be prevented (Table 9.1).

- Approximately 1.5% of people aged over 50 years would be exposed to levels of folic acid intake greater than 1 mg/day (Table A7.2).

Fortification at 420 µg/100 g of flour

- The average intake of folic acid of women aged 16-45 years would increase by 351 µg/day, leading to a total folate intake of 555 µg/day (Table 9.1).

- Approximately 40% of women in this age group would have total folate intakes in excess of 600 µg/day.

- It is estimated that 42 NTD-affected births per year would be prevented (Table 9.1).

- Approximately 9% of people aged over 50 years would be exposed to levels of folic acid intake greater than 1 mg/day (Table A7.2).

On scientific, medical and public health grounds, the Committee concluded that universal folic acid fortification of flour at 240 µg/100 g in food products as consumed would have a significant effect in preventing NTD-affected conceptions and births without resulting in unacceptably high intakes in any group of the population.

11. Any fortification policy should be reviewed in light of the prevailing situation, particularly with regard to improving methodology in folate analysis and the emerging scientific knowledge on bioavailability of natural folates and folic acid from foods.

12. Education to maintain high levels of awareness of the relationship between folic acid and NTDs amongst health professionals and the public, particularly in women of childbearing age, should continue (Chapter 9).

13. Owing to individual difference in dietary patterns, even if fortification were introduced, not all women would achieve the expected mean levels of folate intake. Women who could become pregnant should continue to be advised to take a medicinal or food supplement of 400 µg daily (Conclusion 3).

11. References

[1] MRC Vitamin Study Research Group. Prevention of neural tube defects: Results of the Medical Research Council Vitamin Study. *Lancet* 1991; **338**:131-7.

[2] Department of Health. *Folic Acid in the Prevention of Neural Tube Defects*. Letter from Chief Medical and Nursing Officers. PL/CMO(91)11, PL/CNO(91)6. London, 12 August 1991.

[3] DH Expert Advisory Group. *Folic Acid and the Prevention of Neural Tube Defects*. Department of Health, 1992.

[4] Cornel MC, Erickson JD. Comparison of national policies on periconceptional use of folic acid to prevent spina bifida and anencephaly (SBA). *Teratology* 1997; **55**:134-7.

[5] Fleissig A. Unintended pregnancies and the use of contraception: changes from 1984 to 1989. *BMJ* 1991; **302(6769)**:147.

[6] Allaby M. The risks of unintended pregnancy in England and Wales in 1989. *British Journal of Family Planning* 1995; **21**:93-4.

[7] Boushey CJ, Beresford SAA, Omenn GS, Motulsky AG. A quantitative assessment of plasma homocysteine as a risk factor for vascular disease. *JAMA* 1995; **274**:1049-57.

[8] Wald NJ, Watt HC, Law MR, Weir DG, McPartlin J, Scott JM. Homocysteine and Ischemic Heart Disease. Results of a Prospective Study with Implications Regarding Prevention. *Arch Intern Med* 1998; **158**:862-7.

[9] Department of Health. *Nutritional Aspects of Cardiovascular Disease*. Report on Health and Social Subjects 46. London: HMSO, 1994.

[10] Gregory JR, Collins DL, Davies PSW, Hughes JM, Clarke PC. *National Diet and Nutrition Survey: children aged 1½-4½ years. Volume 1: Report of the diet and nutrition survey.* London: HMSO, 1995.

[11] Finch S, Doyle W, Lowe C, Bates CJ, Prentice A, Smithers G, Clarke PC. *National Diet and Nutrition Survey: people aged 65 years and over. Volume 1: Report of the diet and nutrition survey.* London: The Stationery Office, 1998.

[12] Scott JM, Weir DG. Folic acid, homocysteine and one-carbon metabolism: a review of the essential biochemistry. *J Cardiovas Risk* 1998; Vol 5: No. 4.

[13] Kelly P, McPartlin T, Goggins M, Weir DG, Scott JM. Unmetabolised folic acid in serum; acute studies in subjects consuming fortified food and supplements. *Am J Clin Nut* 1997; **65(6)**:1790-5.

[14] Manzoor M, Runcie J. Folate-responsive neuropathy: report of 10 cases. *BMJ* 1976; **1**:1176-8.

[15] Hoffbrand AV, Newcombe BFA, Mollin DL. Method of assay of red cell folate activity and the value of the assay as a test for folate deficiency. *J Clin Path* 1966; **19**:17-28.

[16] Lavoie A, Tripp E, Hoffbrand AV. The effect of vitamin B_{12} deficiency on methyl folate metabolism and pteroyl polyglutamate synthesis in human cells. *Clin Sci Mol Med* 1974; **4**:617-30.

[17] Savage DG, Lindebaum J. Neurological complications of acquired cobalamin deficiency: clinical aspects. In: Bailliere's Clinical Haematology. Bailliere Tindall: 657-678, 1995.

[18] Stabler SP, Marcell PD, Podell ER, Allen RH, Savage DG, Lindenbaum J. Elevation of total homocysteine in the serum of patients with cobalamin or folate deficiency detected by capillary gas chromatography-mass spectrometry. *J Clin Invest* 1988; **81(2)**:466-74.

[19] Frosst P, Blom HJ, Milos R *et al.* A candidate genetic risk factor for vascular disease: a common mutation in methylenetetrahydrofolate reductase. *Nature Genet* 1995; **10**:111-3.

[20] Arruda VR, von Zuben PM, Chiaparini LC, Annichino-Bizzacchi JM, Costa FF. The mutation Ala677→Val in the methylene tetrahydrofolate reductase gene: a risk factor for arterial disease and venous thrombosis. *Thromb Haemost* 1997; **77**:818-21.

[21] Deloughery TG, Evans A, Sadeghi A *et al.* Common mutation in methylenetetrahydrofolate reductase: correlation with homocysteine metabolism and late-onset vascular disease. *Circulation* 1996; **94**:3074-8.

[22] Department of Health. *Dietary Reference Values for Food Energy and Nutrients for the United Kingdom.* Report on Health and Social Subjects 41. London: HMSO, 1991.

[23] Department of Health and Social Security. *Recommended Daily Amounts of Food Energy and Nutrients for Groups of People in the United Kingdom.* Report on Health and Social Subjects 15. London: HMSO, 1979.

[24] Commission of the European Communities. Nutrient and energy intakes for the European Community. Reports of the Scientific Committee for Food (31st series). Luxembourg: Office for Official Publications of the European Communities, 1993.

[25] Institute of Medicine. A Report of the Standing Committee on the Scientific Evaluation of Dietary Reference Intakes and its Panel on Folate, Other B Vitamins, and Choline and Subcommittee on Upper Reference Levels of Nutrients (pre-publication copy). National Academy Press, Washington D.C. 1998.

[26] Council Directive 79/112/EEC (OJ No L33, 8.2.79).

[27] Council Directive 90/496/EEC (OJ No L275, 6.10.90).

[28] Ministry of Agriculture, Fisheries and Food. *National Food Survey 1998.* London: TSO, 1999.

[29] Sauberlich HE, Kretsch MJ, Skala JH *et al.* Folate requirement and metabolism in nonpregnant women. *Am J Clin Nutr* 1987; **46**:1016-28.

[30] Cuskelly GJ, McNulty H, Scott JM. Effect of increasing dietary folate on red-cell folate: implications for prevention of neural tube defects. *Lancet* 1996; **347**:657-9.

[31] Pfeiffer CM, Rogers LM, Bailey LB, Gregory III JF. Absorption of folate from fortified cereal-grain products and of supplemental folate consumed with or without food determined by using a dual-label stable-isotope protocol. *Am J Clin Nutr* 1997; **66**:1388-97.

[32] Gregory J, Foster K, Tyler H, Wiseman M. *The Dietary and Nutritional Survey of British Adults.* London: HMSO, 1990.

[33] Ministry of Agriculture, Fisheries and Food. *The Dietary and Nutritional Survey of British Adults – Further Analysis*. London: HMSO, 1994.

[34] National Diet and Nutrition Survey: Young people aged 4-18 years. Volume 1: report of the diet and nutrition survey (in preparation).

[35] Mills A, Tyler H. *Food and Nutrient Intakes of British Infants aged 6-12 months*. London: HMSO, 1992.

[36] Rogers I, Emmett P, Baker D, Golding J and the ALSPAC Study Team. Financial difficulties, smoking habits, composition of the diet and birthweight in a population of pregnant women in the South West of England. *Eur J Clin Nutr* 1998; **52**:251-60.

[37] Rogers IS, Emmett P. Diet during pregnancy in a population of pregnant women in the South West of England. *Eur J Clin Nutr* 1998; **52**:246-50.

[38] Mathews F, Yudkin P, Neil A. Folates in periconceptional period: are women getting enough? *Br J Obs Gynae* 1998; **105**:954-59.

[39] Mathews F, Yudkin P, Neil A. Maternal nutrition in pregnancy: an important environmental influence on birth and placental weights at term? *BMJ* 1999; **319(7206)**:339-43.

[40] Health Education Authority. Changing Preconceptions. Volume 2. The HEA Folic Acid Campaign 1995-1998. Research Report, 1998.

[41] Tucker KL, Selhub J, Wilson PW, Rosenberg IH. Dietary intake pattern relates to plasma folate and homocysteine concentrations in the Framingham Heart Study. *J Nutr* 1996; **126(12)**:3025-31.

[42] British National Formulary No 38. British Medical Journal and The Royal Pharmaceutical Society, September 1999.

[43] Foster K, Lader D, Cheesbrough S. Infant Feeding 1995. London: TSO, 1997.

[44] Bates CJ, Mansoor MA, vd Pols J, Prentice A, Cole TJ, Finch S. Plasma total homocysteine in a representative sample of 972 British men and women aged 65 and over. *Eur J Clin Nut* 1997; **51**:1-7.

[45] Homocysteine Lowering Trialists' Collaboration. Lowering blood homocysteine with folic acid based supplements: meta-analysis of randomised trials. *BMJ* 1998; **316**:894-8.

[46] Ward M, McNulty H, McPartlin J, Strain JJ, Weir DG, Scott JM. Plasma homocysteine, a risk factor for cardiovascular disease, is lowered by physiological doses of folic acid. *QJ Med* 1997; **90(8)**:519-24.

[47] Brouwer IA, van Dusseldorp, Thomas CMG, Duran M, Hantvast JGAJ, Eskes TKAB, Steegers-Theunissen RPM. Low dose folic acid supplementation decreases plasma homocysteine concentrations: a randomised trial. *Am J Clin Nutr* 1999; **69**:99-104.

[48] Malinow MR, Duell PB, Hess DL, Anderson PH, Kruger WD, Phillipson BE, Gluckman RA, Block PC, Upson BM. Reduction of plasma homocyst(e)ine levels by breakfast cereal fortified with folic acid in patients with coronary heart disease. *New Engl J Med* 1998; **338(15)**:1009-15.

[49] Schorah CJ, Devitt H, Lucock M, Dowell AC. The responsiveness of plasma homocysteine to small increases in dietary folic acid: a primary care study. *Eur J Clin Nutr* 1998; **52**:407-11.

[50] Daly S, Mills JL, Molloy AM, Conley M, Lee YJ, Kirke PN, Weir DG, Scott JM. Minimum effective dose of folic acid for food fortification to prevent neural-tube defects. *Lancet* 1997; **350**:1666-9.

[51] Creasy M, Alberman ED. Congenital malformations of the central nervous system in spontaneous abortions. *J Med Genet* 1976; **13**:9-16.

[52] McFadden DE, Kalousek DK. Survey of neural tube defects in spontaneously aborted embryos. *Am J Med Genet* 1989; **32**:356-8.

[53] Shaw GM, Lamer EJ, Wasserman CR, O'Malley D, Tolarova MM. Risks of orofacial clefts in children born to women using multivitamins containing folic acid periconceptionally. *Lancet* 1995; **346**:393-6.

[54] Hayes C, Werler MM, Willet WC, Mitchell AA. Case-control study of periconceptional folic acid supplementation and oral clefts. *Am J Epid* 1996; **143(12):** 1229.

[55] Hook EB, Czeizel AE. Can terathanasia explain the protective effect of folic acid supplementation on birth defects? *Lancet* 1997; **350**:513-5.

[56] Czeizel AE, Dudás I. Prevention of the first occurrence of neural-tube defects by periconceptional vitamin supplementation. *New Engl J Med* 1992; **327**:1832-5.

[57] Schorah CJ, Smithells RW, Seller MJ. Terathanasia, folic acid and birth defects. *Lancet* 1997; **350**:1323.

[58] de Onis M, Villar J, Gulmezoglu M. Nutritional interventions to prevent intrauterine growth retardations: evidence from randomized controlled trials. *Eur J Clin Nutr* 1998; **52:S1** S83-93.

[59] Hibbard ED, Smithells RW. Folic acid metabolism and human embryology. *Lancet* 1965; i:1254.

[60] National Congenital Anomaly System. Office for National Statistics.

[61] Murphy M, Whiteman D, Hey K, O'Donnell M, Stone D, Botting B, Schorah C, Wild J, Jones N. Dietary folate and the prevalence of neural tube defects in the British Isles: the past two decades. *Br J Obs Gynae*; in press.

[62] Morris JK, Wald NJ. Quantifying the causes of the decline in the birth prevalence of neural tube defects. *J Med Screen*; in press.

[63] Seller MJ, Nevin NC. Periconceptual vitamin supplementation and the prevention of neural tube defects in South-East England and Northern Ireland. *J Med Genet* 1984; **21(5):** 325-30.

[64] Hall MH. Folic acid deficiency and congenital malformations. *J Obs Gynae Brit Commonwealth* 1973; **79**:159-61.

[65] Smithells RW, Sheppard S, Schorah CJ. Vitamin deficiencies and neural tube defects. *Arch Dis Child* 1976; **51**:944-50.

[66] Yates JRW, Ferguson-Smith MA, Shenkin A, Guzman-Rodriguez R, White M, Clark BJ. Is disordered folate metabolism the basis for the genetic predisposition to neural tube defects? *Clin Genet* 1987; **31**:279-87.

[67] Molloy AM, Kirke P, Hillary I, Weir DG, Scott JM. Maternal serum folate and vitamin B$_{12}$ concentrations in pregnancies associated with neural tube defects. *Arch Dis Child* 1985; **60**:660-5.

[68] Mills JL, Toumilehto J, Yu KF, Colman N, Blaner WS, Koskela P, Rundle WE, Forman M, Toivanen L, Rhoads GG. Maternal vitamin levels during pregnancies producing infants with neural tube defects. *J Pediatr* 1992; **12**:863-71.

[69] Kirke PN, Molloy AM, Daly LE, Burke H, Weir DG, Scott JM. Maternal plasma folate and vitamin B_{12} are independent risk factors for neural tube defects. *QJ Med* 1993; **86**:703-8.

[70] Mills JL, McPartlin JM, Kirke PN, Lee YJ, Conley MR, Weir DG, Scott JM. Homocysteine metabolism in pregnancies complicated by neural-tube defects. *Lancet* 1995; **345**:149-51.

[71] Wald NJ, Hackshaw AK, Stone R, Sourial NA. Blood folic acid and vitamin B_{12} in relation to neural tube defects. *Br J Obs Gynae* 1996; **103**:319-29.

[72] Laurence KM, James N, Miller MH, Tennant GB, Campbell H. Increased risk of recurrence of pregnancies complicated by fetal neural tube defects in mothers receiving poor diets, and possible benefit of dietary counselling. *BMJ* 1980; **281**:1592-4.

[73] Vergel RG, Sanchey LR, Heredero BL, Rodriguez PL, Martinez AJ. Primary prevention of neural tube defects with folic acid supplementation: Cuban experience. *Prenat Diagn* 1990; **10**:149-52.

[74] Smithells RW, Sheppard S, Schorah CJ, Seller MJ, Nevin NC, Harris R, Read AP, Fielding DW. Possible prevention of neural-tube defects by periconceptional vitamin supplementation. *Lancet* 1980; **i**:339-40.

[75] Holmes-Siedle M, Lindenbaum RH, Galliard A, Bobrow M. Vitamins and neural tube defects. *Lancet* 1982; **i**:276.

[76] Smithells RW, Sheppard S, Wild J, Schorah CJ. Prevention of neural-tube defect recurrences in Yorkshire: Final Report. *Lancet* 1989; **2**:498-9.

[77] Seller MJ, Nevin NC. Prevention of neural tube defect recurrences (letter). *Lancet* 1990; **335(8682)**:178-9.

[78] Berry RJ, Zhu L, Erickson JD, Song L, Moore CA, Wang H, Mulinare J, Zhao P, Wong L-YC, Gindler J, Hong S-X, Correa A for the China-US Collaborative Project for Neural Tube Defect Prevention. Prevention of Neural-Tube Defects with Folic Acid in China. *New Engl J Med* 1999; **341**:1485-90.

[79] Wald NJ. Folic acid and the prevention of neural tube defects (unpublished).

[80] Smithells RW, Nevin NC, Seller MJ *et al.* Further experience of vitamin supplementation for the prevention of neural tube defect recurrences. *Lancet* 1983; **i**:1027-31.

[81] Wald N. Folic acid and the prevention of neural tube defects. Maternal nutrition and pregnancy outcome. Eds: Keen CI, Bendich A, Willhite CC. *Ann NY Acad Sci* 1993; **678**:112-29.

[82] Wald NJ. Folic acid and neural tube defects: the current evidence and implications for prevention. In: Neural tube defects (CIBA Foundation Symposium 181). Wiley, Chichester, 1994. 192-211.

[83] Laurence KM, James N, Miller MH, Tennant GB, Campbell H. Double-blind randomised controlled trial of folate treatment before conception to prevent recurrence of neural tube defects. *BMJ* 1981; **282**:1509-11.

[84] Kirke PN, Daly LE, Elwood JH. A randomised trial of low dose folic acid to prevent neural tube defects. *Arch Dis Child* 1992; **67**:1442-6.

[85] Winship KA, Cahal DA, Weber JCP, Griffin JP. Maternal drug histories and central nervous system anomalies. *Arch Dis Child* 1984; **59**:1052-60.

[86] Mulinaire J, Cordero JF, Erickson D, Berry RJ. Periconceptional use of multivitamins and the occurrence of neural tube defects. *JAMA* 1988; **260**:3141-5.

[87] Mills JL, Rhoads GG, Simpson JF, Cunningham GC, Conley MR, Lassman MR, Walden ME, Depp RO, Hoffman HJ and The National Institute of Child Health and Human Development Neural Tube Defect Study Group. The absence of a relationship between the periconceptional use of vitamins and neural tube defects. *N Eng J Med* 1989; **321**:430-5.

[88] Milunsky A, Jick H, Jick S, Bruell CL, MacLaughlin DS, Rotham KL, Willett W. Multivitamin/folic acid supplementation in pregnancy and neural tube defects. *JAMA* 1989; **262**:2847-52.

[89] Werler MM, Shapiro S, Mitchell AA. Periconceptional folic acid exposure and risk of occurrent neural tube defects. *JAMA* 1993; **269**:1257-61.

[90] Bower C, Stanley FJ. Periconceptional vitamin supplementation and neural tube defects: evidence from a case-control study in Western Australia and a review of recent publications. *J Epidemiol Comm Health* 1992; **46**:157-61.

[91] Wald NJ, Law M, Jordan R. Folic acid food fortification to prevent neural tube defects. *Lancet* 1998; **351**:834.

[92] Gallagher PM, Meleady R, Shields DC, Tan KS, McMaster D, Roger R, Evans A, Graham IM, Whitehead AS. Homocysteine and risk of premature coronary heart disease. *Circulation* 1996; **94**:2154-8.

[93] Jacques PF, Bostom AG, Williams RR, Ellison RC, Eckfeldt JH, Rosenberg IH, Selhub J, Rosen R. Relation between folate status, a common mutation in methylenetetrahydrofolate reductase, and plasma homocysteine concentrations. *Circulation* 1996; **93(1)**:7-9.

[94] Alfthan G, Aro A, Gey F. Plasma homocysteine and cardiovascular disease mortality. *Lancet* 1997; **349**:397.

[95] Malinow MR, Nieto FJ, Szklo M, Chambless LE, Bond GS. Carotid artery intimal-medial wall thickening and plasma homocyst(e)ine in asymptomatic adults: the Atherosclerosis Risk in Communities Study. *Circulation* 1993; **87**:1107-13.

[96] Selhub J, Jacques PF, Bostom AG, D'Agostino RB, Wilson PWF, Belanger AJ, O'Leary DH, Wolf PA, Schaeffer EJ, Rosenberg IH. Association between plasma homocysteine concentrations and extracranial carotid-artery stenosis. *N Engl J Med* 1995; **332**:286-91.

[97] den Heijer M, Koster T, Blom HJ, Bos GMJ, Briët E, Reitsma PH, Vandenbroucke JP, Rosendaal FR. Hyperhomocysteinemia as a risk factor for deep-vein thrombosis. *N Engl J Med* 1996; **334**:759-62.

[98] Danesh J, Lewington S. Plasma homocysteine and coronary heart disease: systematic review of published epidemiological studies. *J Cardiovas Risk* 1998; **5**:229-232.

[99] Ratnoff OD. Activation of Hageman factor by L-homocystine. *Science* 1968; **162**:1007-9.

[100] Rodgers GM, Kane WH. Activation of endogenous factor V by a homocysteine-induced vascular endothelial cell activator. *J Clin Invest* 1986; **77**:1909-16.

[101] Rodgers GM, Conn MT. Homocysteine, an atherogenic stimulus, reduces protein C activation by arterial and venous endothelial cells. *Blood* 1990; **75**:895-901.

[102] Celermajer DS, Sorensen K, Ryalls M, Robinson J, Thomas O, Leonard JV, Deanfield JE. Impaired endothelial function occurs in systemic arteries of children with homozygous homocystinuria but not in their heterozygous parents. *J Am Coll Cardiol* 1993; **22**:854-8.

[103] van den Berg M, Boers GH, Franken DG *et al*. Hyperhomocysteinaemia and endothelial dysfunction in young patients with peripheral arterial occlusive disease. *Eur J Clin Invest* 1995; **25**:176-81.

[104] Perry IJ, Refsum H, Morris RW, Ebrahim SB, Ueland PM, Shaper AG. Prospective study of serum total homocysteine concentration and risk of stroke in middle-aged men. *Lancet* 1995; **346**:1395-8.

[105] Malinow MR, Ducimetiere P, Luc G, Evans AE, Arveiler D, Cambien F, Upson BM. Plasma homocyst(e)ine levels and graded risk for myocardial infarction: findings in two populations at contrasting risk for coronary heart disease. *Atherosclerosis* 1996; **126**:27-34.

[106] Obeid OA, Mannan N, Perry G, Iles RA, Boucher BJ. Homocysteine and folate in healthy east London Bangladeshis. *Lancet* 1998; **352**:1829-30.

[107] Bottiglieri T, Crellin RF, Reynolds EH. Folates and neuropsychiatry. In: Folate in Health and Disease. Ed. L Bailey. Marcel Dekker, 1995.

[108] Reynolds EH. Neurological aspects of folate and vitamin B_{12} metabolism. In: Clinics in Haematology 5. Hoffbrand AV, ed. Eastbourne: WB Saunders: 661-96, 1976.

[109] Botez MI, Reynolds EH, eds. Folic Acid in Neurology, Psychiatry and Internal Medicine. New York: Raven Press, 1979.

[110] Shorvon SD, Carney MWP, Chanarin I, Reynolds EH. The neuropsychiatry of megaloblastic anaemia. *BMJ* 1980; **281**:1036-42.

[111] Healton EB, Savage DG, Brust JCM, Garrett TJ, Lindenbaum J. Neurologic aspects of cobalamin deficiency. *Medicine* 1991; **70**:229-45.

[112] Crellin R, Bottiglieri T, Reynolds EH. Folates and psychiatric disorders. *Drugs* 1993; **45**:623-36.

[113] Godfrey PSA, Toone BK, Carney MWP, Flynn TG, Bottiglieri T, Laundy M, Chanarin I, Reynolds EH. Enhancement of recovery from psychiatric illness by methylfolate. *Lancet* 1990; **336**:392-5.

[114] Halsted CH. Water-soluble vitamins. Human Nutrition and Dietetics, 9th edition, 1996. Edited by JS Garrow, WPT James: Churchill Livingstone.

[115] Mortensen PB, Kolvraa S, Christensen E. Inhibition of the glycine cleavage system: hyperglycinemia and hyperglycinuria caused by valproic acid. *Epilepsia* 1980; **21(6)**:563-9.

[116] Clarke R, Smith AD, Jobst KA, Refsum H, Sutton L, Ueland PM. Folate, vitamin B_{12} and serum total homocysteine levels in confirmed Alzheimer disease. *Arch Neurol* 1998; **55**:1449-55.

[117] Schwartz SO, Kaplan SR, Armstrong BE. The long-term evaluation of folic acid in the treatment of pernicious anemia. *J Lab Clin Med* 1950; **35**:894-8.

[118] Wagley PF. Neurologic disturbances with folic acid therapy. *New Eng J Med* 1948; **238**:11-15.

[119] Will JJ, Mueller JF, Brodine C, Kiely CE, Friedman B, Hawkins VR, Dutra J, Vilter RW. Folic Acid and Vitamin B$_{12}$ in Pernicious Anemia. Studies on patients treated with these substances over a ten-year period. *J Lab & Clin Med* 1959; **53(1)**:22-38.

[120] Israels MCG, Wilkinson JF. Risk of neurological complications in pernicious anaemia treated with folic acid. *BMJ* 1949; **2**:1072-5.

[121] Scott E. The prevalence of pernicious anaemia in Great Britain. *J of Coll of Gen Pract* 1960; **3**:80-4.

[122] Chanarin I. The Megaloblastic Anaemia. Second Edition. Blackwell Scientific Publications, Oxford, 1979.

[123] Chanarin I. The Megaloblastic Anaemias. Blackwell Scientific Publications, Oxford, 1990.

[124] Carmel R. Prevalence of undiagnosed pernicious anaemia in the elderly. *Arch Intern Med* 1996; **156**:1097-100.

[125] Brönstrup A, Hages M, Prinz-Langenohl R, Pietrzik K. Effects of folic acid and combinations of folic acid and vitamin B-12 on plasma homocysteine concentrations in healthy, young women. *Am J Clin Nutr* 1998; **68**:1104-10.

[126] Oakley GP Jr. Let's increase folic acid fortification and include vitamin B-12 [Editorial]. *Am J Clin Nutr* 1997; **65**:1889-90.

[127] Herbert V, Bigaouette J. Call for endorsement of a petition to the Food and Drug Administration to always add vitamin B-12 to any folate fortification or supplement. *Am J Clin Nutr* 1997; **65**:572-3.

[128] Giovanucci *et al.* Multivitamin use, folate and colon cancer in women in the nurses' health study. *Ann Intern Med* 1998; **129**:517-24.

[129] Department of Health. *Nutritional Aspects of the Development of Cancer*. Report on Health and Social Subjects 48. London: TSO, 1998.

[130] Editorial. Risk and the inadequacy of science. *Nature* 1997; **385**:1.

[131] Department of Health. *Communicating about Risks to Public Health: Pointers to Good Practice*. London: TSO, 1998.

[132] Keirse MJNC. Changing practice in maternity care. *BMJ* 1998; **317**:607.

[133] White C. Banking on interest. *BMJ* 1998; **317**:607.

[134] Daly LE, Kirke PN, Molloy A, Weir DG, Scott JM. Folate levels and neural tube defects: implications for prevention. *JAMA* 1995; **274**:1698-702.

[135] Daly S, Mills J, Molloy A, Kirke P, Scott J. Folic acid food fortification to prevent neural tube defects. *Lancet* 1998; **351**:834-5.

Annex 1

Recommendations of the report "Folic Acid and the Prevention of Neural Tube Defects"[1]

To prevent recurrence of neural tube defect in the offspring of women or men with spina bifida themselves, or with a history of a previous child with neural tube defect.

1   all such women and men should be counselled about the increased risk of a future offspring being affected;

2   folic acid supplements at a daily dose of 5 milligrams (5000 micrograms) should be advised for all those women who wish to become pregnant or who are at risk of becoming pregnant; the daily dose should be reduced to 4 milligrams (4000 micrograms) if this preparation becomes available as a licensed product;

3   prescriptions of folic acid, when given for the prevention of NTD, should be free of charge;

4   folic acid supplementation should continue until the twelfth week of pregnancy;

5   folic acid-only preparations are preferable to multivitamin preparations;

6   women in this group who are also receiving anticonvulsant therapy need individual counselling by their doctor before starting folic acid supplementation.

To prevent first occurrence of neural tube defect

7   extra folate/folic acid is recommended for all women prior to conception and during the first twelve weeks of pregnancy;

8   the three possible ways of achieving an extra intake of folate/folic acid (eating more folate rich foods, eating foods fortified with folic acid, taking folic acid as a medicinal/food supplement) are not mutually exclusive;

9   women who are planning a pregnancy should eat more folate-rich foods and avoid over-cooking them;

10 the range of breads and breakfast cereals fortified with folic acid should be increased (including wholemeal breads);

11 fortification of foods with folic acid should be restricted to breads and breakfast cereals;

12 the present levels of folic acid fortification in breads and breakfast cereals should not be greatly exceeded;

13 foods which have folic acid added should where practicable indicate the level of fortification;

14 there should continue to be a choice of unfortified breads and breakfast cereals;

15 all women who are planning a pregnancy should be advised to take 0.4 milligrams (400 micrograms) folic acid as a daily medicinal or food supplement from when they begin trying to conceive until the twelfth week of pregnancy;

16 women who have not been supplementing their folate/folic acid intakes and who suspect they may be pregnant should start supplementation at once and continue until the twelfth week of pregnancy;

17 consideration should be given to making folic acid tablets or capsules available free of charge as a pre-pregnancy supplement.

Concerning education, monitoring and review of these recommendations

– there should be major programmes of education for professionals and for the general population;

– there should be a central co-ordination facility to monitor the prevalence of neural tube defects both before antenatal diagnosis and at birth, to determine changes in prevalence and to monitor for early warnings of hazard;

– research should be undertaken on the mechanisms by which folate/folic acid prevents neural tube defects;

– the efficacy of the recommendations in this report should be reviewed formally taking note of the outcomes of future prevention trials.

[1] Department of Health. Folic Acid and the Prevention of Neural Tube Defects. Report from an Expert Advisory Group. 1992. (Available from Department of Health, P O Box 410, Wetherby LS23 7LN.)

Annex 2

Folic Acid Campaign

Health Education Authority, England

Summary

Following the publication of the Medical Research Council's Vitamin Study in 1991, an expert advisory group was set up by the Chief Medical Officers of the UK to review the available evidence relating to folic acid and its role in preventing neural tube defects (NTDs). Its report, *Folic Acid and the Prevention of Neural Tube Defects*, made recommendations for practical action to reduce the incidence of neural tube defects such as spina bifida. Despite widespread dissemination of this report and its recommendations to health professionals, Department of Health research (1995) confirmed the findings of various studies; namely, that women's knowledge of folic acid remained very low.

This prompted the Department of Health to commission the Health Education Authority (HEA) to run a £2.3m national integrated campaign aimed at increasing the average daily intake of folates and folic acid in women who might become pregnant by at least 400 µg from foods containing natural folate, foods fortified with folic acid and folic acid supplements. This campaign ran from autumn 1995 to spring 1998; however, the HEA has continued to promote folic acid advice as part of the work of the Food and Nutrition Programme. The objectives of the work are to:

- increase awareness of the importance of taking *additional* folic acid before conception and 12 weeks into pregnancy in the general female population and in influential professional groups;

- increase the availability of fortified breads and breakfast cereals;

- increase the number and availability of appropriate supplements, especially those that are licensed; and

- make fortified products and supplements more easily identifiable.

Women are advised to increase their daily intake of folic acid by 400 µg by:

- eating more folate-rich foods;

- eating more foods fortified with folic acid – especially breads and breakfast cereals; and

- the commercial sector, including food retailers and manufacturers, trade associations, and manufacturers of ovulation predictor and pregnancy testing kits.

Health professionals and women planning pregnancy (the core target group) were the key audiences for the campaign's work in its first year. In the second year, the campaign began to position folic acid as a general women's health issue, and broadened its work to target all women of childbearing age, to encompass "future planners" – women not currently planning to have a baby, who would probably do so at some time in the future. Young people, as the parents of tomorrow, were a key focus of work in the third year.

A critical element of the work was to create partnerships with the voluntary, public and commercial sectors, at local and national levels, in order to influence and increase the effectiveness of the campaign. Health professionals have been integral to the success of the work. A range of strategies was adopted to convey different messages to various audiences and to influence the behaviour of professionals and the public. Elements of the work were designed to reinforce one another and included:

- developmental research, literature reviews, monitoring surveys, policy analysis;

- public and professional information – leaflets, posters, advertising, public relations, media work;

- supporting local innovation in various sectors;

- collaboration with health professional bodies;

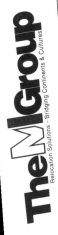
- developing a folic acid flash labelling scheme for foods (especially breads and breakfast cereals) fortified with folic acid;

- producing the Folic Acid Education Pack for secondary school teachers, containing guidance on how folic acid advice can be given to pupils as part of core curriculum subjects and Personal, Social and Health Education;

- joint promotions with retailers and trade associations such as the National Association of Master Bakers.

These interventions have helped to create a positive climate of change, intended to make women more aware of folic acid, more likely to see information about it, more able to buy it easily, and more likely to take it.

Results

The campaign was underpinned by an extensive programme of research at all stages of its planning, execution and evaluation, focusing primarily on the public, health professionals and the commercial sector. Quantitative research and other indicators used to track the campaign's progress found that:

- spontaneous (unprompted) awareness of folic acid among women of childbearing age had increased from 9% (1995) to 49% (1998);

- prompted awareness among women of childbearing age had risen from 51% (1995) to 89% (1998);

- the percentage of women claiming to take folic acid when trying for a baby had risen from 24% of (recently) pregnant women in 1997 to 38% in 1998; the percentage of women claiming to take folic acid during the first twelve weeks of pregnancy had risen from 54% of (recently) pregnant women in 1997 to 68% in 1998;

- 71% of health professionals spontaneously identified folic acid as "very important" for women planning a pregnancy in 1997 – compared with 64% in 1996;

- 49% of health professionals who had seen campaign information claimed to have changed their practice as a result;

- the range of fortified products and supplements had increased (18 companies were currently signed up to the folic acid flash labelling scheme – representing over 250 products);

- the number of licensed 400 µg folic acid supplements had doubled;

- the number of unlicensed 400 µg folic acid supplements had increased from 9 in May 1996 to 18 in March 1998.

- prescription rates for folic acid had increased.

Issues and challenges

The campaign faced a number of significant challenges. As fortification of grain products is voluntary, not mandatory, industry was initially reluctant to take action in this area. There was low awareness of folic acid advice among the target population, and an estimated 30 to 50% of pregnancies in England and Wales is unplanned. The notion of making preconceptional health changes was new to many women, and neural tube defects are rare conditions, which needed to be made real to women in order to motivate them to take folic acid.

With regard to women themselves, key considerations include: their low awareness of folic acid; the off-putting nature of the term "acid"; the fact that folic acid offers a deferred benefit; the need to convey technical information; the prevailing climate of confusion/suspicion over new dietary information; and the sensitive nature of the subject.

Conclusions

The campaign has achieved heartening increases in awareness of folic acid, and encouraging levels of claimed supplement use among recently pregnant women. However, folic acid advice in England relies on women taking voluntary action to ensure that they are taking sufficient levels of extra folic acid. Women who plan pregnancy are therefore the only group that can be expected to take a supplement at the appropriate time for reducing the risk of neural tube defects, as a supplement is only advised at the stage of planning pregnancy, and not as something all women of childbearing age should be taking.

Of the 38% of recently pregnant women who took folic acid preconceptionally (1998 tracking survey), 65% had planned their pregnancy. Women who do not plan their pregnancies therefore remain one of the groups that is hardest to reach, as are those who, for whatever reason, have not received the relevant health promotion advice, or are unable to understand or relate to it. The widespread adoption of the folic acid flash labelling scheme, and the greater availability of folic acid supplements and foods fortified with folic acid show what can be achieved within a voluntary framework by working closely with the commercial sector and legislative bodies.

However, reaching women who have unplanned pregnancies via the dietary route requires health professionals and others to give folic acid advice to all women of childbearing age. Ultimately, this relies on women's own active choices and changes in behaviour for success: an enormous challenge.

Annex 3

Folic acid: dietary sources, analysis and food composition data

Dietary Sources and Forms

Folic acid (pteroylmonoglutamic acid, PGA) occurs in food as a range of folate vitamers, which differ in the extent of the reduction of the pteroyl group, the presence of one-carbon substituents and the number of glutamyl residues attached to the pteroyl group. Folic acid is also the normal form used for fortification purposes because of its greater stability and lower cost. The most abundant forms found are 5-methyltetrahydrofolates (5-MTHF), 5- and 10-formyltetra-hydrofolates, and 5,6,7,8-tetrahydrofolic acid. Monoglutamates and polyglutamates of 5-MTHF are widely distributed in foods, whereas formyl forms tend to be found in foods of animal origin. The main dietary sources of folic acid are cereal and cereal products (especially fortified breads and breakfast cereals), leafy green vegetables and milk products.

Folate Analysis and Speciation in Food

At present, the most widely used and accepted procedure for food folate analysis is the microbiological assay (MA) using *Lactobacillus rhamnosus* (formerly *Lactobacillus casei*) as the test organism[1], where a response of the organism to the mixture of folates present is measured. Even with the development of semi-automated procedures including the microtitration plate format[2], the MA is both time-consuming and demanding in execution. Additionally, the response of the organism to the different folate forms is not always identical. At pH 6.8 for organism growth and 0-1 ng assay range, the growth response of *Lactobacillus rhamnosus* to 5-MTHF was less than the growth of PGA (the normal folate used to calibrate the assay), but at pH 6.2 the growth response to these two forms is almost identical[3].

Preliminary enzymatic deconjugation is essential in order to measure the polyglutamated folate forms. The conditions of this deconjugation need to be optimised for individual foods, especially in the choice of the deconjugase enzyme, pH and length of incubation. The conditions of the MA used are critical for precision, and a further drawback is that the different vitamers are not measured individually. Typical values obtained from recent European intercomparison studies suggest that the within-laboratory variation for the MA is around 10%, and the between-laboratory variation is 20-30%, depending on the foods analysed[4].

High-performance liquid chromatography (HPLC) with either UV detection (PGA only) or fluorescence (reduced folates) detection has been developed[5,6]. Results from EU method intercomparison studies show that there can be problems with losses during sample extraction and clean-up, peak identification and calibration. Currently, only 5-MTHF can be quantified with any degree of certainty. Typical values for within- and between-laboratory variation for the HPLC determination of 5-MTHF in foods are about 5-10% and 15%, respectively[7,8].

Radio-protein binding assays ('radioassays', RPBA) have also been used for folate analysis in foods but variable results have been obtained and are not currently recommended for food use[4]. Alternatively, enzyme protein-binding assays based on the 96-well microtitration plate format have been used for total folate determinations, and comparable results have been obtained with the MA[9,10]. Enzyme-linked immunosorbent assays (ELISAs) using various antibody preparations have also been applied to the determination of specific folate vitamers with some success (Finglas *et al.*, unpublished results). More recently, antibody-based techniques have been used in a biosensor instrument for the determination of folic acid (and 5-MTHF) in fortified foods. Initial results compared favourably with HPLC values but were lower than the microbiological data[11].

The development of food certified reference materials (CRMs) will greatly assist in the quality control of folate measurements. Four CRMs have been produced (a milk powder, a wholemeal flour, a lyophilised mixed vegetable material, and a lyophilised pigs' liver material) and certified for total folate by MA and 5-MTHF by HPLC, and these are now available from the Institute for Reference Materials and Measurements (IRMM), Geel, Belgium[12].

Folate Analysis in Biological Tissues and Fluids

The determination of folate in biological tissues and fluids is usually undertaken using MA, RPBA and HPLC procedures. In serum, 5-MTHF is the main folate vitamer present in its monoglutamate form. In erythrocyctes, 5-MTHF is also the predominant form, but is present mainly as polyglutamates.

The main problem with the use of the radioassay kits is the choice of the pH because PGA (the normal calibrant used in the kit) and 5-MTHF exhibit different pH-dependent affinity binding curves with the milk folate binding protein[13]. Equal affinity between both forms is found at pH 9.3 and therefore this is the pH of choice in most kits. However, small differences in assay pH may strongly affect the results. Typical values obtained from recent European intercomparison studies for folate determinations in serum and whole blood using MA and various radioassay kits give between-laboratory variation of about 30 and 40%, respectively. The variation for MA (whole blood only) was lower at about 25%[14]. Similar results have also been reported for serum and whole blood folate using MA , RPBA and HPLC methods[15]. The same authors found two- to nine-fold differences in folate concentrations between methods, with the greatest variation occurring at critical low concentrations.

Some concern has also been expressed that the current extraction procedures for the determination of erythrocyte folate need re-evaluation. Published literature suggests that increased deoxy-hemoglobin (which can bind folate electrostatically) yields more assayable folate by MA, and increased oxy-hemoglobin (which cannot bind red cell folate) yields less assayable folate[16]. In addition, there has also been some debate as to the most appropriate procedure for the determination of erythrocyte folate. Significant differences in folate values have been obtained in individuals with homozygous (TT) MTHFR variant using MA and RPBA procedures[17]. It has been further postulated that the folate form in these individuals may have an increased response in the RPBA assay compared with the assay calibrant, giving erroneous higher values.

HPLC procedures for folate analysis in blood use both fluorometric and electrochemical detection[18]. More recently, a stable isotope dilution gas chromatography-mass spectrometry (GC-MS) procedure was reported for the quantitation of red blood cell folate using bacterial synthesised $^{13}C_6$-labelled folate as an internal standard[19]. This type of approach gives high sensitivity, specificity and accuracy/precision, and may be suitable as a reference procedure in the future.

These results demonstrate the need for developing and validating reference methods for serum and whole blood analyses for folate, and for properly characterised reference materials. Although there are several commercial plasma and whole blood preparations available for use as quality control materials, mainly for RPBA procedures, they have not been analysed by other procedures. Recently, the First International Standard for Whole Blood Folate analysis was released by the National Institute for Biological Standards and Control for use with MA and RPBA procedures.

Folate Data in Food Composition Databases and Tables

Much of the folate data in the current UK food tables (McCance & Widdowson's The Composition of Foods, 5th edition)[20] is based on the microbiological procedure. In the future, HPLC data on 5-MTHF, and possibly other folates, may be included as supplemental tables.

The average daily folate intake calculated using 4th edition of the McCance & Widdowson's Composition of Foods[21] was about 50% lower compared with daily intakes calculated using the 5th edition[20] (Finglas et al)[22]. This is because the 4th edition substantially underestimates the folate content of foods rich in 5-MTHF[21,23]. The 5th edition contains revised folate data for several food groups using improved microbiological procedures and in the same study, calculated folates intakes based on the more recent edition, were about 20% lower than intakes based on analyses of duplicate diets. Folate data for a wide range of foods (especially vegetables, cereals and meats) in the 5th edition are currently being updated for inclusion in the 6th edition which is to be published in late 2000.

A comparison of folate data in seven national food composition tables in Europe have been undertaken for a range of similar foods. There was a 2-3 fold variation in total folate obtained by microbiological assay in vegetables, milk and bread. HPLC values were also given for total folate in various liver samples in one set of tables and these values were considerably higher (10-fold) than the corresponding microbiological data. There was no obvious explanation for these differences, but they may be due to differences in sampling or methods of analysis used. Further work is investigating these variations and attempting to establish an 'Expert System' for evaluating the quality of folate data appearing in food composition tables.

References

[1] Keagy PM. Folacin - microbiological and animal assays. In: *Methods of Vitamin Assay* (4th Edition), eds. J. Augustin, B.P. Klein, D.A. Becker & P.B. Venugopal, 1985. John Wiley & Sons, New York, pp.445-96.

[2] Newman EW Tsai JF. Microbiological analysis of 5-formyltetrahydrofolic acid and other folates using an automatic 96-well plate reader. *Anal Biochem* 1986; **154**, 509-15.

[3] Wright AJA, Phillips DR. The threshold growth response of *Lactobacillus casei* 5-methyltetrahydrofolic acid: implications for folate assays. *Br J Nutr* 1985; **53**, 569-73.

[4] Finglas PM, Faure U, Southgate DAT. First BCR-intercomparison on the determination of folates in food. *Food Chem* 1993; **46**, 199-213.

[5] Gregory LF, Sartain DB, Day BPF. Fluorometric determination of folacin in biological materials using high performance liquid chromatography. *J Nutr* 1984; **114**, 341-53.

[6] Witthöft C, Bitsch I. HPLC methods to analyse folate patterns in food and in human plasma as a precondition to evaluate availability of food folates by biokinetic methods. In: *Bioavailability '93, Proceedings Part 2*, Ed. U. Schlemmer, Bundesforschungsanstalt für Ernährung, Karlsruhe, 1993; pp. 436-9.

[7] Vahteristo L, Finglas PM, Witthöft C, Wigertz K, Seale R, de Froidmont-Görtz I. Third EU MAT intercomparison study on folate analysis using HPLC procedures. *Food Chem* 1996; **57 (1)**, 109-11.

[8] Finglas PM, Wigertz K, Vahteristo L, Witthoft C, Southon S, de Froidmont-Goertz I. Standardisation of HPLC procedures for the determination of naturally-occurring folates in food. *Food Chem* 1998; **64**, 245-55.

[9] Finglas PM, Faulks RM, Morgan MRA. The development and characterisation of a protein-binding assay for the determination of folate - potential use in food analysis. *J Micronutr Anal* 1988; **4**, 295-308.

[10] Finglas PM, Kwiatkowska C, Faulks RM, Morgan MRA. Comparison of a non-isotopic, microtitration plate folate-binding assay and a microbiological method for the determination of folate in raw and cooked vegetables. *J Micronutr Anal* 1988; **4**, 309-322.

[11] Bostrom M, Finglas PM, Persson B, Wahlstrom L. Determination of folate by BiacoreQuant in two milk-based food reference materials: SRM 1846 and CRM 421. Proc. 112th AOAC Annual Meeting & Exposition, 13-17 September, 1998. Montreal, Canada.

[12] Finglas PM, Scott KJ, Witthoft C, van den Berg H, de Froidmont-Goertz I. The certification of the mass fractions of vitamins in four reference materials: wholemeal flour (CRM 121), milk powder (CRM 421), lyophilized mixed vegetables (CRM 485) and lyophilized pig's liver (CRM 487), 1998b. EUR-report 18320. Luxembourg: Office for Official Publications of the European Communities, 1999.

[13] Givas JK, Gutcho S. pH Dependence of the binding of folates to milk binder in radioassay of folates. *Clin Chem* 1975; **21**, 427-8.

[14] van den Berg H, Finglas PM, Bates C. FLAIR intercomparisons on serum and red cell folate. *Int J Vitam Nutr Res* 1994; **64**, 288-93.

[15] Gunter EW, Bowman BA, Caudill SP, Twite DB, Adams MJ, Sampson EJ. Results of an international round robin for serum and whole blood folate. *Clin Chem* 1996; **42 (10)**, 1689-94.

[16] Wright AJA, Finglas PM, Southon S. Erythrocyte folate analysis: a cause for concern ? *Clin Chem* 1998;, **44 (9)**, 1886-91.

[17] Molloy AM, Mills JL, Kirke PN, Whitehead AS, Wier DG, Scott JM. Whole-blood folate values in subjects with different methylenetetrahydrofolate reductase genotypes: differences between radioassay and microbiological assays. *Clin Chem* 1998; **44**, 186-88.

[18] Lucock M, Green M, Hartley R, Levene MI. Physicochemical and biological factors influencing methylfolate stability: use of dithiothreitol for HPLC analysis with electrochemical detection. *Food Chem* 1993; **47**, 79-86.

[19] Santhosh-Kumar CR, Deutsch JC, Hassell KL, Kolhouse NM, Kolhouse JF. Quantitation of red blood cell folates by stable isotope dilution gas chromatography-mass spectrometry utilizing a folate internal standard. *Anal Biochem* 1995; **225**, 1-9.

[20] Holland B, Welch AA, Unwin ID, Buss D, Paul AA, Southgate DAT. McCance and Widdowson's The Composition of Foods, 5th Edition, 1991; Cambridge: RSC/MAFF.

[21] Paul AA, Southgate DAT. McCance and Widdowson's The Composition of Foods, 4th edition, 1978; HMSO, London.

[22] Finglas PM, Southon S, Wright AJA, Bailey AL, Belsten JL. Comparison of calculated micronutrient intake with analysed intake obtained by direct analysis of duplicate diets. Proc. 1st International Conference on Dietary Assessment Methods, 20-23 September, 1992, Minneapolis St Paul, USA. *Amer J Clin Nutr* 1992, **59**, 286S.

[23] Finglas PM, Wright AJA, Faulks RM, Southgate DAT. Revised folate content of UK vegetables - implications for intake. In: *Recent knowledge on iron and folate deficiencies in the world,* Eds. S. Hercberg, P. Galan & H. Dupin, Colloque INSERM, 1990; **197**, 385-92.

Annex 4

Morphogenesis of the neural tube in humans

Normal neural tube formation Neural tube formation is a complex multistep process. In terms of gross morphology, neurulation begins with induction of the neural plate, observed as the thickening of the ectodermal cells that constitute the neural plate, first observed around day 18 after conception. This is followed progressively by the shaping of the neural plate, its bending by elevation of the neural folds and their over-arching, and finally their fusion in the midline. This closure process starts at the hindbrain/cervical junction at around day 21 and proceeds in a very specific manner, and is completed with closure of the cephalic portion around day 24 and the posterior neuropore around day 26. This produces the neural tube down to the level of the future upper sacral region, and constitutes primary neurulation. Subsequently, the most distal part of the neural tube is extended subcutaneously by the aggregation of cells - a process termed secondary neurulation.

In molecular terms, the formation of the neural tube begins much earlier, with pattern formation, the molecular mapping of the basic body plan. Details of this are still being discovered, but it appears that around day 15 after conception, when the embryo is at the early gastrula stage, a small group of around 125-150 cells in the immediate vicinity of the node or organiser is marked out as neural precursor cells: those nearest the node will form the brain, and those most distant the spinal cord. Numerous genes are involved in controlling the subsequent patterning of the developing neural tube and its shaping and bending and also, it is believed, its closure. The evidence for the latter is that there are five separate closure sites involving specific regions along the neuraxis in a particular sequence, which result in the completed primary neurulation (multisite closure).

Neural tube defects Overall, neural tube defects are considered to occur because there is failure of closure of the neural tube, either in a localised region or throughout its length. The precise region involved defines the type of neural tube defect - spina bifida, anencephaly or encephalocele. There are a number of mouse models for neural tube defects and the cause is known to be either mutations of single genes or the effects of several genes acting together. In addition, a multifactorial aetiology can be demonstrated in some mouse models with both genes and environmental agents contributing to the cause.

Needs of the neurulating embryo Obviously, neural tube formation is associated with rapid cell proliferation. Not only is the neural plate enlarging, but, as the neural folds elevate, the underlying mesoderm is expanding. At the same time, the entire embryo is growing and other organs such as the heart and gut are also forming. Thus, there is an excessive demand for precursors and co-factors for the macromolecules needed for all this morphogenesis, and these necessarily are supplied by the mother.

Nutrition of the embryo At the time of formation of the neural tube, the mature chorioallantoic placenta, which is commonly associated with fetal nutrition, does not exist. At the commencement of neurulation and through to day 21-22, the sole source of embryonic nutrition is by way of the histiotroph. This is a rich mixture derived from secretions of the uterine glands, which accumulates in spaces in the syncytiotrophoblast. This is digested by the cytotrophoblast, and nutrients diffuse across to the embryo. Then, in the middle of the process of neurulation, around day 21-22, intermittent pulsation of the paired heart tubes begins and the definitive haemotrophic type of nutrition is initiated. In this, nutrients from the maternal blood cross the villus barrier to the fetal blood and are carried around the developing body by the heart and blood circulatory system. However, for the remainder of neural tube formation, the two types of nutrition are concurrent.

Annex 5

NTD affected pregnancies in the United Kingdom

	England and Wales (1998[1])	Scotland (1997[2])	Northern Ireland (1998[3])
Number of live births	635,549	57,940	24,277
Number of NTD affected live births[4]:	**68**	**66**	**14***
Spina bifida	54**	}	
Anencephaly	8	}66	
Encephalocele	6	}	
Number of still births	3,401	319	132
Number of NTD affected still births[4]:	**26**	**8**	
Spina bifida	9	}	
Anencephaly	14***	}8	
Encephalocele	3***	}	
Number of therapeutic abortions	177,871[5]	12,109[6]	-
Number of NTD affected therapeutic abortions[4]:	**305**	**59[7]**	
Spina bifida	120	17	
Anencephaly	163	28	
Encephalocele	22	1	

* including still births, ** includes one child with spina bifida occulta, *** includes one child with anencephaly and encephalocele

[1] (TSO, 1999a)

[2] (ISD (Scotland) CSA, Edinburgh, unpublished data)

[3] (DHSS Northern Ireland, unpublished data)

[4] (National Congenital Anomaly System)

[5] (TSO, 1999b)

[6] (Notification (to the Chief Medical Officer, SODoH) of abortions performed under the Abortion Act 1967)

[7] Includes hydrocephalous, craniorachischisis, holoprosencephaly, Arnold-Chiari syndrome, and other congenital malformations of the spinal cord

Annex 6

Models to estimate the impact of hypothetical folic acid fortification of flour on folate intakes in the UK

The data used for all calculations were derived from the UK government-sponsored dietary surveys: Dietary and Nutritional Survey of British Adults[1], National Diet and Nutrition survey (NDNS) of children aged 1½ to 4½ years[2], NDNS of people aged 65 and over[3] and the NDNS of young people aged 4 to 18 years[4]. These were based on randomly drawn, nationally representative samples of individuals, each of whom was asked to complete a weighed dietary record over a consecutive 4-day or 7-day period. To minimise seasonal bias, entry of respondents into each study was spread over a full year. No attempt was made to correct for possible bias due to non-response or under-reporting of food intake.

Table 1 summarises key properties of the survey data underlying the dietary intake calculations.

Table 1   Key features of the dietary surveys used to model intakes of folic acid

Survey	Year	Respondents	Response rate	Number of days
Adults (16 – 64 yrs)	1986/7	2197	70%	7
1½ to 4½ yrs	1992/3	1675	81%	4
65 yrs & over	1994/5	1275	59%	4
Young (4 – 18 yrs)	1997/8	1701	64%	7

In each survey, a nutrient database, comprising several thousand foods, was used to translate daily records of foods consumed into estimated intakes of folate (the sum of naturally occurring folate and added folic acid). The 1994/5 food composition table was applied to all surveys at or before this date for those foods where it was clear that the definition had not changed between surveys. It is possible that slightly greater accuracy might have been achieved by retrospective application of the 1997/8 nutrient look-up table in estimating intakes from NDNS of young people aged 4-18 years.

In fortification programmes recently implemented in the USA and Hungary, cereal grains (USA) and bread (Hungary) have been used as the vehicles for folic acid. Modelling undertaken by the COMA Working Group originally considered the likely impact on folate intakes if one or more of the following three staple foods were fortified with folic acid: flour, breakfast cereals, milk. However, preliminary calculations suggested that only flour was worth studying in more detail because of its near universal consumption.

The first step was to compute the amount of flour in any given food product in the nutrient database. This was simplified by assuming that the proportion for flour was constant within each food group. However, it varied between groups according to the approximate values given in Table 2.

Table 2   Assumed flour content (% weight) of 11 distinct groups of flour-containing products

Food group	% Flour
Pizza	30
"Other" cereals	25
White bread	75
Wholemeal bread	75
Soft grain bread	75
"Other" bread	72
Biscuits	50
Fruit pies	22
Buns, cakes & pastries	45
Sponge type puddings	10
"Other" puddings	10

The flour content of food groups not represented in Table 2 was assumed to be zero, which may introduce a slight downward bias into estimates of the impact of folic acid fortification of flour. However, a small bias in the opposite direction could result from the fact that approximately 1% of flour consumed in the UK is derived from imported products and would therefore escape any mandatory fortification scheme implemented in the UK.

Data from Table 2 were used to compute folate intakes based on individual consumption of different flour products. For example, if flour is fortified at the rate of 140 μg of folic acid per 100 g, then an individual consuming 200 g of white bread on a given day would be expected to take in an extra 210 μg of folic acid (140 * 0.75 * 200/100 μg) as a result of fortification.

Estimation of folic acid intakes in Table A7.1 required a distinction to be drawn between naturally occurring folate and synthetic folic acid. It was assumed that the total folate content listed in food composition tables consisted entirely of natural folate for all but the following foods: soft grain bread (40% of the total folate assumed to be folic acid), wholegrain/high-fibre breakfast cereals (50% of the total folate assumed to be folic acid), other breakfast cereals (80% assumed to be folic acid) and dietary supplements (100% folic acid). Hypothetical mandatory fortification of flour was assumed to be entirely in the form of folic acid and not at all in the form of natural folate.

The most demanding modelling problem was to reconcile the fact that interest lies in estimation of habitual intakes of folate and folic acid whereas data are available only from short-run, consecutive-day, weighed food intake diaries. Such data will tend to exaggerate variability in intakes between individuals unless seasonal, weekly or day-to-day variations can be extricated from true between-person variation. Evidence from NDNS surveys suggests that, when mean daily folate intake is assessed from 4- or 7-day weighed diaries, day-to-day variation inflates the apparent between-person standard deviation of the intake distribution by about 7-10%. The contribution of variation over longer timescales (e.g. seasonal) is almost certainly no greater than this. A possible mechanism for undoing the distension of the intake distribution caused by within-person variation components has been described by Gay[5]. Unfortunately, this mechanism was found inappropriate for distributions of folate intake owing to skewness introduced by a minority of NDNS respondents who took folic acid supplements. Therefore, it could only be applied safely when considering folate intake derived from food sources only.

The net effect of the assumptions underlying the assessment of the impact of hypothetical folic acid fortification scenarios is unlikely to be large: potential biases operate in different directions and may, in large degree, cancel one another out. The greatest distortion of estimated distributions of folate intake is likely to lie in overly extreme estimates of extreme intakes, resulting from inability to compensate for within-person components of variation. However, some attempt was made to estimate its magnitude and it was felt that this distortion did not influence the conclusions drawn from the modelling exercise.

References

[1] Gregory JR, Foster K, Tyler H, Wiseman M. *The Dietary and Nutritional Survey of British Adults*. London: HMSO, 1990.

[2] Gregory JR, Collins DL, Davies PSW, Hughes JM, Clarke PC. *The National Diet and Nutrition Survey of children aged 1½ to 4½ years*. London: HMSO, 1995.

[3] Finch S, Doyle W, Lowe C, Bates CJ, Prentice A, Smithers G, Clarke PC. *National Diet and Nutrition Survey: people aged 65 years or over*. Volume 1: Report of the diet and nutrition survey. London: HMSO, 1998.

[4] National Diet and Nutrition Survey: Young people aged 4-18 years. Volume 1: Report of the diet and nutrition survey (in preparation).

[5] Gay C. Estimation of population distributions of habitual nutrient intake based on a short-run weighed food diary. *Brit J Nutr* (in press).

Annex 7

Table A7.1 A model to display mean daily intakes* of folic acid (µg/day) derived from the fortification of flour by age group according to different strategies for universal fortification of flour

Age group and sex	Current intake* Mean total (natural folate + folic acid) intake (µg)			Calculated intakes Mean daily folic acid intake at different flour fortification levels including folic acid provided by the current voluntary fortification of foods and dietary supplements				
	Natural folate µg	Folic acid µg	Total intake µg	140 µg/ 100 g	200 µg/ 100 g	240 µg/ 100 g	280 µg/ 100 g	420 µg/ 100 g
1½-4½ y M + F[1]	107	20	127	82	108	126	144	206
11-14 y F[2]	175	36	211	145	192	224	255	365
15-18 y F[2]	189	26	215	137	185	217	249	360
16-45 y F[3]	186	19	204	136	186	219	253	370
50-64 y M[3]	283	21	304	205	283	336	388	572
50-64 y F[3]	206	17	223	143	197	233	269	395
65y+ M[4]	232	36	268	186	251	294	337	488
65y+ F[4]	181	33	214	143	191	223	254	365

* All intake values calculated on the basis of the food and supplement intake patterns recorded at the time of the diet and nutrition survey fieldwork, but using, in common, a 1995 version of MAFF's nutrient databank for levels of folates in foods except for 11 – 14 and 15 – 18 yr olds, for which 1997 data were used. Since fieldwork for those aged 16 – 64 yr was over 10 years ago, data about how often supplements were being taken in 1986/7 cannot be taken to reflect current levels of folic acid supplement taking.

Table A7.2 The impact of different levels of universal fortification of flour with folic acid on the distribution of total folate intake (natural folate and folic acid) for various population groups

Age group and sex	Current intake of food folate + folic acid μg/day	140μg/100g of flour ≤600 μg	140μg/100g >1000μg Inc supp#	140μg/100g >1000μg Exc supp#	200μg/100g ≤600 μg	200μg/100g >1000μg Inc supp	200μg/100g >1000μg Exc supp	240μg/100g ≤600 μg	240μg/100g >1000μg Inc supp	240μg/100g >1000μg Exc supp	280μg/100g ≤600 μg	280μg/100g >1000μg Inc supp	280μg/100g >1000μg Exc supp	420μg/100g ≤600 μg	420μg/100g >1000μg Inc supp	420μg/100g >1000μg Exc supp
		Percentage of population with total (folate and folic acid) daily intakes (%)														
1½–4½ M + F*1	126	100	0	0	100	0	0	100	0	0	99.8	0	0	98.5	0	0
11-14 F**2	211	98.7	0	0	95.8	0	0	92.9	0	0	87.4	0	0	66.5	0.4	0
15-18 F**2	215	98.1	0	0	96.7	0	0	92.1	0	0	85.5	0	0	60.8	1.4	0
16-45 F*3	204	99.3	0	0	97.2	0.1	0	93.0	0.1	0	87.0	0.1	0	60.4	1.1	1.0
50-64 M*3	304	81.0	0.4	0.4	60.8	0.7	0.7	45.0	2.2	1.8	39.9	5.5	5.1	16.1	25.3	25.3
50-64 F*3	223	98.9	0	0	95.1	0	0	90.5	0.3	0.3	82.7	0.3	0.3	54.1	1.4	1.4
65+ M*4	268	91.8	0	0	80.1	0.5	0.2	66.3	0.8	0.2	58.4	1.1	0.5	31.5	10.4	9.8
65+ F*4	214	97.4	0.5	0	95.7	0.5	0	94.3	0.5	0	89.9	0.5	0	67.3	2.2	0.9
Average of 50+ age group with intakes	-	92.3	0.23	0.1	82.9	0.43	0.23	74.0	0.95	0.58	67.7	1.85	1.47	42.2	9.83	9.35

* Intakes based on 1995 food composition values
** Intakes based on 1997 food composition values
# Including or excluding dietary supplements

100

References

[1] Gregory JR, Collins DL, Davies PSW, Hughes JM, Clarke PC. *The National Diet and Nutrition Survey of children aged 1½ to 4½ years*. London: HMSO, 1995.

[2] National Diet and Nutrition Survey: Young people aged 4-18 years. Volume 1: report of the diet and nutrition survey (in preparation).

[3] Gregory JR, Foster K, Tyler H, Wiseman M. *The Dietary and Nutritional Survey of British Adults*. London: HMSO, 1990.

[4] Finch S, Doyle W, Lowe C, Bates CJ, Prentice A, Smithers G, Clarke PC. *National Diet and Nutrition Survey: people aged 65 years or over*. Volume 1: Report of the diet and nutrition survey. London: HMSO, 1998.

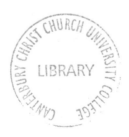

Printed in the United Kingdom for The Stationery Office
J99825 C15 01/00 9385 11746

101